S0-BNW-488

HANDBOOK
OF
PEDIATRIC MEDICAL EMERGENCIES

HANDBOOK OF PEDIATRIC MEDICAL EMERGENCIES

By

ADOLPH G. DeSANCTIS, M.D.

Professor of Pediatrics and Chairman of the Department of Pediatrics, Post-Graduate Medical School, New York University-Bellevue Medical Center; Director of Pediatrics, University Hospital, New York University-Bellevue Medical Center; Director of Pediatrics, Gouverneur Hospital, New York City

and

CHARLES VARGA, M.D.

Instructor in Pediatrics, Post-Graduate Medical School, New York University-Bellevue Medical Center; Assistant Attending Pediatrician, University Hospital, New York University-Bellevue Medical Center; Assistant Visiting Pediatrician, Gouverneur Hospital, New York City

WITH FIFTY-ONE ILLUSTRATIONS

ST. LOUIS

THE C. V. MOSBY COMPANY

1951

Reprinted July, 1951
Reprinted April, 1952

Printed in the
United States of America

Press of
The C. V. Mosby Company
St. Louis

CONTRIBUTORS

Alfred B. Amler, M.D.

Nathan Cabot, M.D.

Adolph G. DeSanctis, M.D.

James Dick, M.D.

James F. Johnson, M.D.

Robert F. Kinberger, M.D.

Vincent de Paul Larkin, M.D.

Thomas F. X. Lenihan, M.D.

Harold R. Mancusi-Ungaro, M.D.

Joseph F. Raffetto, M.D.

William P. Riley, M.D.

Samuel C. Southard, M.D.

Charles Varga, M.D.

PREFACE

The material in this handbook was prepared over a period of years to serve as a guide for members of the resident staff and for physicians enrolled in the courses offered by the Pediatric Department of the Post-Graduate Medical School. It was our purpose to include conditions encountered in pediatric practice which call for rapid, emergency therapy. It was certainly not intended that this be a complete text of pediatrics, and for this reason certain problems have not been included. In addition, in order to make the material practical we have endeavored to present therapy only. Nevertheless, as we progressed we realized that in certain situations basic review of important symptoms, signs, or criteria might simplify diagnosis of the less common conditions and thereby facilitate early treatment. We proceeded, therefore, along these lines. Finally, after several revisions a small handbook was completed and printed privately for general distribution.

It was extremely gratifying that the demand for the privately printed edition has been sufficiently great so that a more complete revision has become necessary. At the suggestion of several outstanding pediatricians we undertook such a revision. Furthermore, it was felt that a short section on pediatric procedures commonly employed might be of additional value.

Pediatricians in other institutions may have various other methods of therapy for certain disorders. The methods herein outlined are those which have generally been used with good results.

References have been made to the standard pediatric journals and to textbooks of pediatrics. Only those specific references are generally included which we felt would be of actual value in aiding the physician in the outline of therapy.

Several of the contributors to the privately printed edition have not continued in their original capacity because of changes in geographic location or because other duties have prevented their cooperation with us in this book. Nevertheless, because of their efforts with the original handbook we again extend our thanks to them. They are: Clarence W. Harwood, M.D., Paul Rousseau, M.D., Flora F. Silberbush, M.D., Pasquale A. Statile, M.D., and Alma M. Sullivan, M.D.

We wish to express our appreciation to all of the contributors to the present volume. We wish also to acknowledge the cooperation of Dr. Benjamin Daversa of the Department of Obstetrics of the Fitkin Memorial Hospital, Neptune, New Jersey, for his valuable suggestions in the preparation of the section on management of resuscitation in the newborn.

We extend our thanks also to Miss Florence M. DePew, nurse in charge of Babies' Ward of the University Hospital, and members of her staff for their suggestions and cooperation in the preparation of the illustrations.

The line drawings were prepared by Mr. James J. States. His willing cooperation made the problem an easy one.

The photographs were taken on Babies' Ward of the University Hospital by Dr. Nathan Cabot.

Finally, the secretarial duties in the preparation of the manuscript have been excellently performed by our departmental secretary, Mrs. Virginia States Anlian. We extend our sincere thanks to her.

ADOLPH G. DESANCTIS, M.D.
CHARLES VARGA, M.D.

New York City

CONTENTS

CHAPTER VII

PAGE

CHAPTER VIII

CHAPTER IX

CHAPTER X

ADDENDA

APPENDIX

LIST OF ILLUSTRATIONS

LIST OF TABLES

CHAPTER I

CARDIOVASCULAR EMERGENCIES

Certain cardiac emergencies may occur in infancy and childhood. All of them require prompt diagnosis and therapy. Signs and symptoms associated with cardiac failure may be noted. Particular emphasis, however, should be placed on a rapid respiratory rate (30 to 40 per minute or higher) and liver engorgement (the liver may extend to the level of the umbilicus). In addition to these, dyspnea and fine moist rales in the lung fields (especially at the bases) may be present. Symptoms of shock may occasionally develop. (See page 182.)

The prompt use of digitalis may often be lifesaving in cardiac emergencies. Taussig[1] states that,

> "the indications for the use of digitalis are essentially the same for children as for adults: (1) Cardiac failure, (2) dilatation of the heart and a gallop rhythm, (3) excessively rapid heart action (180-200 beats per minute), (4) the occurrence of the more serious cardiac arrhythmias, namely, auricular fibrillation, auricular flutter, and paroxysmal tachycardia, and (5) occasionally a shunt reversal."

ACUTE CARDIAC FAILURE

Treatment

1. Oxygen in high concentration.*[2]
2. Complete bed rest.
3. Sedation for restlessness.
   (a) Barbiturates. Short-acting (Seconal, Nembutal), gr. ½ to gr. 1 rectally or intramuscularly.
   (b) Morphine sulfate. Generally, the dosage suggested in the section on Preanesthetic Medication may be adequate (see page 176).

---

*A brief illustrated section on oxygen therapy is included in Chapter X, page 217 et seq.

ACUTE CARDIAC FAILURE—Cont'd
Treatment—Cont'd

4. Digitalis.
   (a) Total initial digitalization.
      (1) *Rapid-acting digitalis glycosides* when immediate action is desirable. Various glycosides are favorites in different parts of the world. Those generally available with recommended dosage in children are presented in Table I.

TABLE I. CARDIAC GLYCOSIDES

CARDIAC GLYCOSIDE	TRADE NAME	MANUFACTURER	DOSAGE FOR TOTAL DIGITALIZATION
1. Digitoxin	Digitalline nativelle Purodigin Crystodigin Digitoxin	Fougera (Varick) Wyeth Lilly Squibb; Abbott; Parke-Davis	Digitoxin group 0.01 mg. per pound. Either orally, intravenously, or intramuscularly
2. Digoxin	Digoxin	Burroughs-Wellcome	*Orally* 0.014 to 0.033 mg. per pound *I.M. or I.V.* 0.005 to 0.007 mg. per pound
3. Lanatoside A, B, C*	Digilanid	Sandoz	0.01 mg. per pound orally, I.M. or I.V.
4. Strophanthin*	Strophoside K Strophanthin	Sandoz Abbott	0.005 to 0.007 mg. per pound, I.V.
5. Ouabain* (Strophanthus gratus)	Ouabain	C. D. Smith; Lilly; Burroughs-Wellcome; Hynson	0.003 to 0.006 mg. per pound, I.V. (One-half of the total dose may be given initially followed by 1/10 of the total dose every ½ hour until the entire amount has been given

*The glycosides most commonly used in this country are digitoxin and digoxin. The other preparations are listed mainly because foreign physicians or clinics may use them preferentially either because of individual familiarity or local availability. Lanatoside C (Cedilanid—Sandoz) has been *eliminated* from this book because Taussig[1] states that it has a narrow margin of safety.

It must be remembered that children react differently to various dosages. It is best to start with low doses and increase them gradually until the desired effect is achieved. It cannot be emphasized too strongly that when using digitalis preparations careful attention must be paid to the status of the individual—including special cardiac and EKG studies. It must be emphasized, however, that an EKG is generally only of real aid if an EKG was also done prior to digitalization.

ACUTE CARDIAC FAILURE—Cont'd
Treatment—Cont'd
4. Digitalization—Cont'd
(a) Total initial digitalization—Cont'd

(2) *Slow-acting digitalis leaf.* Dose 1/6 gr. (0.01 Gm. of powdered leaf) per pound of body weight. Regardless of which preparation of digitalis is used, the dose can be calculated from the above by knowing the exact value of the preparation in grains or grams. In the event in which rapid digitalization is necessary, give one-half of the 24-hour dose immediately, and the remaining digitalis should be divided into four doses every 6 hours, e.g., an 80-pound child will require 0.8 Gm. of digitalis. Give 0.4 Gm. stat and the remaining 0.4 Gm. must be divided into four doses, thus giving 0.1 Gm. every 6 hours. (1½ gr. equals 1 cat unit).

5. Diuretics.
   (a) *Aminophylline.* Rectally, intramuscularly, or intravenously; 6 mg. per kilogram of body weight (children under 45 kilograms of body weight).
   (b) *Mercurials.* 0.5 to 1.0 c.c. every second or third day, as needed.

ARRHYTHMIAS

A. PAROXYSMAL AURICULAR TACHYCARDIA

Although the etiology of this condition is not known, prompt treatment is mandatory.

1. Stimulation of the carotid sinus or pressure on the eyeball may occasionally suffice in older children, but digitalis is generally required in infants.
2. In severe cases, a rapid-acting digitalis preparation must be used. (See Table I in section on Acute Cardiac Failure, page 18.)

ARRHYTHMIAS—Cont'd
A. PAROXYSMAL AURICULAR TACHYCARDIA—Cont'd

3. Only in desperate cases in which all other drugs have been proved unsuccessful should ouabain be administered.
4. Quinidine sulfate may give good results in some children. EKG should be done before this drug is administered. It must be administered with extreme caution, however, because some children may react unfavorably. The optimum dosage is 3 mg. per pound every 3 hours given orally. The bitter taste of the medication may be masked by giving it as a 5% suspension in chocolate syrup. If medication cannot be tolerated orally or if the patient cannot take the medication orally, a preparation of quinidine sulfate in propylene glycol is available for intramuscular injection. The same dosage is used as for the oral route.[2a] The medication should be continued until either the abnormal rhythm is abolished or until toxic manifestations develop. The toxic manifestations include nausea, vomiting, diarrhea, and EKG changes. The latter consist mainly of a 40 to 50% prolongation of the QRS time.
5. *Mecholyl* (acetyl-beta-methylcholine), a parasympathicomimetic drug, has been used in doses of 3 to 10 mg. intramuscularly. It may, however, cause heart block. *Atropine sulfate should be kept on hand to counteract excessive parasympathetic stimulation.*
6. *Acetylcholine bromide*[3, 4] may also be useful when digitalis fails. Extreme caution must be used when administering this drug, however, because of its marked action on the cardiac mechanisms. Its pharmacologic antidote, atropine sulfate, must be on hand also as mentioned under Mecholyl above. Dosage: 1.0 mg. may be used as an initial dose intravenously. It is preferable that the heart rate and an EKG be observed while administering this drug. The development of bradycardia or the estab-

lishment of a sinus mechanism indicates that no more drug should be given and that the condition has been brought under control. Because of the rapidity with which Acetylcholine Bromide is destroyed in vivo, the dose (1.0 mg.) may be repeated every 3 or 4 minutes until a result is obtained.

B. HEART BLOCK

1. Congenital. Usually only supportive therapy is necessary.
2. Acquired.
   (a) Due to infection. Existing infection should be treated with specific methods.
   (b) Drug toxicity—such as Mecholyl* (used freely in megacolon treatment) and potassium* (used in treatment of diarrhea).
      (1) Specific pharmacologic antidote.*
      (2) Ephedrine sulfate, 25-50 mg.
      (3) Supportive therapy.

C. AURICULAR FIBRILLATION

Although rare in infancy, this arrhythmia may occur in older children with mitral disease.

Digitalization. (See section on Digitalis in Cardiac Failure, page 18.)

D. AURICULAR FLUTTER

This is a relatively rare condition in infancy and childhood. Generally, the diagnosis is made by EKG findings.

Treatment

1. Prompt digitalization as outlined previously.

---

*See special sections on Drug Poisoning, pages 139 and 140.

ARRHYTHMIAS—Cont'd

E. VENTRICULAR TACHYCARDIA

Marked ventricular tachycardia may occasionally be noted in children as a toxic manifestation of digitalis overdosage. The objective of therapy is to prevent ventricular fibrillation.

Treatment

1. Immediate effect may be achieved by slow intravenous injection of 5 to 10 c.c. of a 10% magnesium sulfate solution.
2. Quinidine sulfate may then be used orally in doses of 1 to 2 gr. every 3 hours for 2 to 3 days.

F. ACUTE CIRCULATORY ARREST

Experience, experimentally with animals and clinically with patients, has shown that sudden circulatory arrest may be due either to cardiac standstill or ventricular fibrillation.

Treatment of Cardiac Standstill[5]

1. 0.2 to 0.3 c.c. of 1:1000 solution of epinephrine hydrochloride DILUTED TEN TIMES WITH STERILE ISOTONIC SALINE injected
   (a) Intracardially or
   (b) Into right jugular vein.
2. Cardiac massage.

Treatment[4] **of Ventricular Fibrillation**

1. Cardiac massage.
2. Intravenous procaine (as outlined under section on Serum Sickness, page 177).

SEVERE PAROXYSMAL DYSPNEA

(Especially as Seen With Tetralogy of Fallot)

Treatment[6]

1. Knee-chest position.
2. Morphine (of specific value). Dose: 1.0 mg. per 5 kilograms of body weight.

PERICARDIAL EFFUSION

The clinical diagnosis is at times very difficult. However, when a child suffers from an acute infectious disease and a sudden embarrassment of the circulation occurs with decrease in intensity of the heart sounds and an increase in cardiac dullness, the possibility of pericardial effusion should be considered. The apical impulse may become feeble, but the pulse remains strong. To confirm the diagnosis, x-ray of the chest should be made and venous pressure taken. The x-ray might reveal an onion-shaped heart with the absence of pulsation of the margins. After the pericardial effusion has persisted for twenty-four to forty-eight hours, there may be a rise in the leukocyte count (over 20,000), an elevation of temperature (over 103°), and a rise in the sedimentation rate. These often persist in spite of improvement of the original infection and will lead to suspicion of pericardial effusion, especially if the venous pressure is increased. Additional findings may include enlargement of the liver and orthopnea.

Criteria for Paracentesis of Pericardium

Only occasionally is there a real need for pericardial tap because the vast majority of pericardial effusions resolve spontaneously.

1. Presence of purulent pericarditis, as evidenced by marked leukocytosis and hyperpyrexia, indicates need for tap.
2. Similarly, increase in size of the cardiopericardial shadow and increase in size of liver indicate cardiac tamponade and requires tap.

Treatment

1. The tamponade of the heart has to be relieved. A paracentesis of the pericardium has to be done. This procedure is outlined in another section (page 216).

TRAUMA

The treatment is usually surgical and supportive.

1. Surgical—repair of wound.
2. Supportive—transfusions, oxygen, sedation (if necessary).

ARTERIAL EMBOLISM AND THROMBOSIS

The occasional occurrence[7] of this condition, especially during the course of septic states, prompts its inclusion in this handbook.

Diagnosis

A. Sudden onset of coldness or pallor, diminution or loss of muscle power, discoloration of skin, lack of pulsation in vessels supplying part—in an extremity which was previously normal.

Note: It is important for therapy to consider (1) the differential diagnosis between arterial spasm and occlusion and (2) the progression of the condition.

1. Generally speaking, the persistence of a diminished blood flow for more than an hour or two is more indicative of occlusion than spasm.
2. (a) Pallor of skin is almost invariably followed in a few hours by a bluish or mottled discoloration.
   (b) If gangrene is to supervene, a line of demarcation will almost certainly appear within 24-48 hours.
   (c) If the arterial occlusion is incomplete or if collateral circulation is sufficient to carry the load, the pallor will gradually disappear (sometimes this takes a week or more) and will be progressively replaced by a more pinkish tint.

Treatment

1. Take immediate precautions to prevent a superimposed or secondary infection locally.
   (a) Cleanse widely with 70% ethyl alcohol.
   (b) Encase in a sterile bandage (change twice daily, using aseptic technique).

ARTERIAL EMBOLISM AND THROMBOSIS—Cont'd
Treatment—Cont'd

2. Avoid application of heat.
3. A period of watchful waiting is indicated unless signs of general toxicity develop.
4. Sympathetic block may be indicated.
5. Antibiotics should be used liberally to control and prevent infection.
6. Surgical consultation is suggested.

CEREBRAL THROMBOSIS IN CONGENITAL HEART DISORDERS

This may be a common, serious complication in patients with congenital malformations of the heart. The usual cause of this complication is polycythemia with associated increase in blood viscosity. Nevertheless, any condition associated with severe anoxemia may precipitate cerebral thrombosis. In any event, an important contributing factor is dehydration.

Signs

1. Although a variety of neurological signs may be present, convulsions and hemiplegia are most generally seen.

Treatment[1]

1. Venisection.
   (a) 100-250 c.c. of blood may be withdrawn from a child 2-6 years of age, depending on age and size of child and height of red blood count.
   (b) Oxygen.
   (c) Intravenous saline, 5% glucose or cross-matched plasma.
2. Continue intravenous fluids for 12-24 hours after venisection.
3. Anticoagulant.
   (a) Intravenous heparin to prolong clotting time 20-30 minutes and maintained thus for 24 hours.

CEREBRAL THROMBOSIS IN CONGENITAL HEART DISORDERS—Cont'd
Treatment—Cont'd
3. Anticoagulant—Cont'd

(b) Heparin, 0.5 mg. per kilogram. Keep adding same amount to 5% glucose in H_2O every hour. (If the coagulation is prolonged excessively, the heparin should be stopped and intravenous glucose administered. Hemorrhagic episodes should be controlled with transfusions).

References

1. Taussig, H. B.: Congenital Malformations of the Heart, New York, 1947, The Commonwealth Fund.
2. Andrews, A. H.: Manual of Oxygen Therapy Technique, Chicago, Ill., 1947, The Year Book Publishers, Inc.
2a. Gold, H.: Quinidine in Disorders of the Heart, New York, 1950, Paul B. Hoeber, Inc.
3. Philipsborn, H. F., and Gibson, S.: Paroxysmal Tachycardia; Report of Two Cases Treated With Acetyl-Choline Bromide, Pediatrics **1:** 205, 1948.
4. Linenthal, E. J., and Freedberg, A. S.: Measures Used in the Prevention and Treatment of Cardiac Arrhythmias, New England J. Med. **241:** 575, 1949.
5. Beecher, H. K., and Linton, R. R.: Epinephrine in Cardiac Resuscitation, J. A. M. A. **135:** 90, 1947.
6. Taussig, H. B.: Tetralogy of Fallot: Especially the Care of the Cyanotic Infant and Child, Pediatrics **1:** 307, 1948.
7. Gross, R. E.: Arterial Embolism and Thrombosis in Infants, Am. J. Dis. Child. **70:** 61, 1945.

CHAPTER II

GASTROINTESTINAL EMERGENCIES

ACUTE TOXIC DIARRHEA

Prompt treatment should be instituted in all cases of diarrhea in infants and young children because of the marked lability of their water- and electrolyte-conserving mechanisms. This is even more true in the premature infant with diarrhea.

Emergency medical attention is especially indicated in the presence of acidosis, dehydration, and shock. Emphasis will be placed on the management of this phase.

For practical purposes, nevertheless, an arbitrary division may be made:

A. Treatment of dehydration, acidosis, and shock.

B. Maintenance of body fluids, electrolytes, and nutrition.

A. Treatment of Dehydration, Acidosis, and Shock

1. Discontinue oral feeding.
2. Take a blood sample for
   (a) CO_2 combining power.
   (b) Typing and cross-matching (include complete studies).
   (c) Complete blood count.
   (d) Hematocrit.
3. Start an intravenous infusion of M/6 sodium lactate at 20 drops per minute. Adjust total amount to be given after the CO_2 combining power is obtained in accordance with the following formula:*

---

*Generalities may be difficult to follow in any one specific case. Caution must be exercised to avoid alkalosis during the administration of alkali, especially when given too rapidly intravenously or in great quantities. Whenever possible, CO_2 combining power and blood pH determinations should be done frequently during the course of alkali therapy. Careful clinical observation of the patient is also necessary. Very frequently, ⅔ of the total calculated amount of alkali is sufficient to re-establish normal CO_2 combining power.

ACUTE TOXIC DIARRHEA—Cont'd
A. Treatment of Dehydration, Acidosis, and Shock—Cont'd

Normal CO_2 (55) – actual $CO_2 \times$ weight in pounds = total amount of diluted solution to be used.*

4. Subsequent alkali therapy.*
   (a) If CO_2 is within normal limits, isotonic saline solution may be used.
   (b) If CO_2 is between 20 and 40 volumes %, continue with M/6 sodium lactate.
   (c) If CO_2 is less than 20 volumes %, use 3.75% sodium bicarbonate.

      Formula:

      1 Gm. of sodium bicarbonate per kilogram of body weight will generally increase the CO_2 by 38 volumes %.
5. Supportive measures.
   (a) Plasma or blood transfusions as indicated.
   (b) Oxygen as indicated.
   (c) Intravenous adrenal cortical extract as recommended in section on Acute Adrenal Insufficiency (page 67).
   (d) Vitamin K—4.8 mg. intravenously or intramuscularly.

---

*In a recent symposium on acidosis and alkalosis,[1] Hartmann has offered the following routine for treatment of acidosis in accordance with the classification of the severity of the acidosis:

Mild acidosis (CO_2 combining power 37.0 to 45.0 volumes %).
1 to 5 c.c. of molar lactate per kilogram per day given orally is usually sufficient.

Moderate acidosis (Co_2 combining power from 25.0 to 37.0 volumes %)
30 c.c. per kilogram of M/6 sodium lactate added to 40 c.c. per kilogram of Ringer's solution usually suffices when given subcutaneously or intravenously.

Severe acidosis (CO_2 combining power 15.5 to 25.0 volumes %)
60 c.c. per kilogram of M/6 sodium lactate added to 40 c.c. per kilogram of hypotonic Ringer's solution given subcutaneously is usually sufficient.

Extreme acidosis (CO_2 combining power less than 15.5 volumes %)
30 c.c. per kilogram of M/6 lactate intravenously in addition to the mixture of sodium lactate in hypotonic Ringer's solution, mentioned in the previous section on severe acidosis.

ACUTE TOXIC DIARRHEA—Cont'd

B. Maintenance of Body Fluids, Electrolytes, and Nutrition

1. *Approximate maintenance requirements* (while diarrhea persists):

Water	150-200 c.c. per kilogram of body weight
Carbohydrate	18-20 Gm. per kilogram of body weight
Protein	3-4 Gm. per kilogram of body weight
Total calories	80-100 calories per kilogram of body weight
NaCl	A total of 1 Gm. per day or more per day depending on NaCl loss in perspiration and stools.

2. After dehydration, acidosis, and shock have been overcome, the following parenteral fluids may be used in any combination to maintain body fluids, electrolytes, and nutrition in accordance with the above maintenance requirements.*
   (a) 5% glucose in isotonic saline alternated with 10% glucose in water, given intravenously.
   (b) 2½% glucose in saline alternated with 2½% glucose in water subcutaneously.
   (c) Protein hydrolysates.
      (1) *Baxter's Travamin*—an enzymatic protein digest from bovine plasma.
      Each liter contains:

Calories	200 Gm.
NaCl	3.0 Gm.
Protein	50.0 Gm.
Protein nitrogen	8.0 Gm.

---

*Several important considerations must be emphasized.

1. There are a variety of available "repair" solutions. The composition of these has been recently presented.[2, 3] A modification of these two presentations is included in Table II.
2. There are certain dangers in electrolyte fluid therapy. These, too, have been succinctly tabulated.[2]

Dangers in Electrolyte and Fluid Therapy

(1) Failure to correct shock because of hemoconcentration.
(2) Early use of subcutaneous glucose which immobilizes fluid and causes further electrolyte deficiency.
(3) Alkalosis and tetany from excessive alkali.
(4) Edema, potassium loss, and increased acidosis from excessive saline.
(5) Potassium intoxication from rapid or excessive K therapy, especially in dehydrated states.
(6) Postacidotic state—excessive deposition of K, HPO_4, and Ca in tissues with fall in serum values.
(7) Intoxication or sloughing from calcium therapy.
(8) Hypoglycemia on stopping long-continued intravenous glucose therapy.

TABLE II. ELECTROLYTE CONTENTS OF REPLACEMENT SOLUTIONS

SOLUTION	1,000 C.C. REPAIR SOLUTION CONTAINS GRAMS/MILLIEQUIVALENTS								
	NaCl	KCl	$CaCl_2$ $2H_2O$	$Mg\ Cl_2$ $2H_2O$	$NaHCO_3$	MOLAR SODIUM LACTATE, C.C.	K_2HPO_4	NH_4Cl	REMARKS
0.9% Saline	9.0/154								1-2 parts may be mixed with 1 part 5-10% glucose
Hartmann's Ringer-Lactate	6.0/103	0.4/5.4	0.2/2.2	0.2/2.4		25/25			1-2 parts may be mixed with 1 part 5-10% glucose
M/6 Sodium Lactate						167/167			60 c.c. (45-60) per kilogram for 30-35 volumes % $BHCO_3$ deficit; may be mixed with 2 pints saline
⅔ Saline ⅓ M/6 Sodium Lactate	6.4/103					56/56			
M/6 $NaHCO_3$ (Isotonic)					14.0/167				Intravenous only; 55 c.c. per kilogram for 30-35 volumes % deficit = 17 ml. of 5% solution
Darrow, 1946	4.0/69	2.7/36				53/53			80 c.c. per kilogram per 24 hr.; then 150 ml. per kilogram of mixture 1 part to 2 parts of 5% glucose per day
Darrow, 1947	3.0/51	2.7/36			4.4/52				Mix 1 part to 2 parts 5-10% glucose given as above
Butler (10% glucose)	0.58/10	0.89/12				20/20	0.25/2.6		150-200 ml. per kilogram at rate of 0.8 ml. per minute for infants per day
M/6 NH_4Cl in Saline 0.9%	9.0/154							0.9/167	As outlined in section on Treatment of Alkalosis (page 46)
Ringer's	8.5/146	9.3/4	0.2/2.2						May be used in accordance with suggestions for physiological saline
Hypotonic Ringer's	6.0/102.7	0.4/5.4	0.2/1.6	0.2/3.8					In accordance with the recommendations in the section on Diabetic Acidosis (page

ACUTE TOXIC DIARRHEA—Cont'd

B. Maintenance of Body Fluids, Electrolytes, and Nutrition—Cont'd

2. Parenteral fluids—Cont'd

(c) Protein hydrolysates—Cont'd

(1) *Baxter's Travamin*—Cont'd

A preparation containing 5% dextrose is also available providing 400 calories per liter.

Intravenously. The preparation containing dextrose is preferable because of its higher caloric value.

Rate: 20 to 30 drops per minute.

Amount: Sufficient to supply required protein intake.

Subcutaneously. The preparation without dextrose is recommended in amounts above.

(2) Mead's Amigen (Each 500 c.c. of Amigen contains 200 calories and 1 Gm. NaCl).

Intravenously. Two parts 5% Amigen with 5% dextrose with 1 part distilled water.

Rate: 20 drops per minute.

Amount: Adjusted to supply requirements as outlined in table on maintenance requirements (page 29).

Subcutaneously. One part 5% Amigen with 5% dextrose to one part distilled water.

Note: Proper maintenance cannot generally be obtained by exclusive subcutaneous administration of fluids. The decrease in concentration of solutions adaptable for subcutaneous use makes it impossible to maintain nutrition without increasing fluid volume to over twice the maintenance requirements.

In addition, fluids may be slowly absorbed from subcutaneous sites. This latter difficulty may be circumvented, however, to a certain extent by the concurrent use of hyaluronidase (Alidase, Searle; Hydase, Wyeth).

ACUTE TOXIC DIARRHEA—Cont'd

B. Maintenance of Body Fluids, Electrolytes, and Nutrition—Cont'd

2. Parenteral fluids—Cont'd

(c) Protein hydrolysates—Cont'd

Note—Cont'd

(1) Start subcutaneous clysis in the usual manner.

(2) Test sensitivity of patient to hyaluronidase by injecting 0.02 c.c. of a prepared solution intradermally. A positive reaction is indicated by a wheal with pseudopods appearing within 5 minutes and lasting 20 to 30 minutes.

(3) In the absence of demonstrable sensitivity, inject 500 viscosity units (1 ampule Alidase—Searle) or 150 T.R. units (1 ampule Hydase—Wyeth) through the wall of the rubber tubing near the hypodermoclysis needle a few minutes after the clysis is started.

(d) *Darrow's solution.**

(1) Treat shock if present as previously outlined.

(2) Administer the KCl-NaCl lactate mixture (percentage composition of which is indicated in Table II, page 30) 80 to 100 c.c. per kilogram of body weight subcutaneously. *Give slowly over a period of at least 4 hours.*

(3) Supplement water intake to 150 to 200 c.c. per kilogram of body weight intravenously using 5 to 10% dextrose in water.

(4) If the frequency of the diarrheal movements decreases, a modified Darrow's solution may be given orally as follows: 1 part KCl-NaCl lactate with 2 parts 5% dextrose with water. The

*Balance studies with infants with severe diarrhea have revealed the need for potassium in many cases. The regime outlined is that suggested by Darrow. Extreme caution must be exercised, however, to avoid the insidious onset of potassium intoxication whenever Darrow's solution is given parenterally. It is suggested that hyaluronidase should not be used when Darrow's solution is used subcutaneously. Should potassium intoxication develop, calcium gluconate is the specific chemical antidote. The exact treatment for potassium intoxication is outlined in the section on Poisoning, page 140.

ACUTE TOXIC DIARRHEA—Cont'd

B. Maintenance of Body Fluids, Electrolytes, and Nutrition—Cont'd

2. Parenteral fluids—Cont'd

(d) *Darrow's solution*—Cont'd

(4) Modified Darrow's solution—Cont'd

total amount thus administered should be 150 c.c. per kilogram per day. If the patient cannot tolerate this amount orally, supplemental parenteral fluids should be administered to maintain hydration.

(5) When oral formula feedings are started, 1 to 2 Gm. of KCl may be added to the total 24-hour formula until the total caloric value of the formula is at least 70 calories per kilogram per day.

C. **Chemotherapy and Antibiotic Therapy**

1. The sulfonamides used in gastrointestinal infections, such as Sulfathalidine, Sulfasuxidine, sulfadiazine, sulfamerazine, or triple sulfas should be used in appropriate dosages.
2. Streptomycin may also be used orally (0.5 Gm. daily) and parenterally (0.5 Gm. per day in divided doses).
3. Aureomycin and Chloromycetin (20-50 mg. per kilogram per day) have proved most effective, depending on the infecting organisms.*

VOMITING

As in diarrhea, emergency treatment is necessary in correcting electrolyte and water imbalance and shock. This again is followed by maintenance of balance of hydration, electrolytes, and nutrition. With vomiting, acidosis or alkalosis may be present; alkalosis from loss of gastric HCl, acidosis from loss of alkaline duodenal content often accen-

*It is well to bear in mind, however, that aureomycin may cause diarrhea when given orally. In addition, recent evidence indicates that a smaller amount of aureomycin is absorbed during diarrhea than during a period when stools are normal.

VOMITING—Cont'd

tuated by low or absent gastric HCl in infants, and the acidosis produced through starvation.

A. If acidosis is present, treat as under Diarrhea (page 27 et seq.).

B. If alkalosis with tetany or impending tetany is present, treat as in diarrhea, but instead of starting Na lactate, start with:*

1. Intravenous calcium chloride 5% solution 1 c.c. per kilogram or calcium gluconate.
2. Ringer's solution
3. Lactate-Ringer's solution.
4. Dilute HCl intravenously for quick response.
5. Breathing of CO_2 and oxygen.

When immediate danger of tetany has subsided, maintain nutrition as in diarrhea.

C. If presence of acidosis or alkalosis cannot be determined clinically, start on lactate-Ringer's solution and await laboratory results.

D. Basic cause of vomiting to be determined and treated as soon as possible.

ACUTE SURGICAL ABDOMEN

The various types of acute surgical abdomen call for certain preliminary tests (in addition to C.B.C. and urinalysis) and treatments.

1. Blood CO_2 and chlorides.
2. Typing and cross-matching (including Rh studies).
3. Intravenous 5% dextrose in saline to re-establish proper hydration and electrolyte balance.
4. Plasma and/or whole blood as needed.
5. Proper preanesthetic medication.
6. Prophylactic chemotherapy and/or antibiotic therapy.

---

*Also refer to section on Alkalosis, page 46.

CORROSIVE POISONS (Lye)
(See Section on Poisoning, page 129)

FOREIGN BODIES IN THE GASTROINTESTINAL TRACT

A. **In Esophagus**

Remove through esophagoscope.

B. **In Stomach**

1. Small, nonsharp (or nonpointed) objects may be allowed to pass through.
   (a) Avoid cathartics, bulky foods, or any change in diet.
   (b) Observe progress every day or every other day by fluoroscope.
2. *Large objects* (over 2 inches in length) or sharp objects (needles, pins, etc.) should be removed by gastroscope.

C. **In Intestine**

Allow to pass through unless stationary for over 4 days. Then, surgical removal may be indicated.

GASTROINTESTINAL HEMORRHAGE

Gastrointestinal hemorrhage is not a common occurrence in infancy or childhood. Nevertheless, its occurrence is certainly an alarming experience.

The common causes for gastrointestinal hemorrhage may be listed as follows:

1. Blood dyscrasias.
2. Congenital malformations of the gastrointestinal tract.
   (a) Meckel's diverticulum.
   (b) Reduplication of the intestine.
3. Intussusception.
4. Intestinal polyps.
5. Peptic ulcers (perforated, especially in the newborn).
6. Varices (esophageal).
7. Pyloric stenosis (a rare cause of bleeding).

GASTROINTESTINAL HEMORRHAGE—Cont'd

8. Toxemias.
9. Hereditary hemorrhagic telangiectasis.

Treatment

The treatment of the hemorrhage is of immediate importance.

1. Adequate sedation of patient is essential.
2. Transfusion with properly typed (including Rh) blood or plasma. (When plasma is used, fresh or lyophilized plasma is preferable.)
3. Vitamin C and vitamin K should be given in usual therapeutic doses parenterally.
4. The use of Thrombin, Topical, in cases of bleeding from the esophagus, stomach, or small intestines may be of real value.[4, 5]
   (a) Administer 10 to 20 c.c. of M/7 phosphate buffer*
   (b) Administer 5,000 to 10,000 N.I.H. units of Thrombin, Topical (Parke-Davis), diluted in 10 to 20 c.c. of M/7 phosphate buffer orally.
   (c) If bleeding is controlled, continue plain buffer solution every half hour for 72 hours.
   (d) Periodic blood CO_2 combining power and blood pH examinations should be made during the use of phosphate buffer solutions in order to avoid disturbance in electrolyte balance.

References

1. Hartmann, A.: Round Table Discussion on Acidosis and Alkalosis, Pediatrics 2: 584, 1948.
2. McBryde, A., et al.: Round Table Discussion on Management of Infantile Diarrhea and Dysentery, Pediatrics 2: 335, 1948.
3. Hand, A. M., and Leininger, C. R.: Parenteral Fluid Therapy in Children, M. Clin. North America 34: 53, 1950.
4. Rogers, T. M.: Management of Gastrointestinal Hemorrhage—Using Topical Thrombin, J. A. M. A. 137: 1035, 1948.
5. Plummer, K.: Hereditary Hemorrhagic Telangiectasis. Intestinal Bleeding: Case Report and Therapy With Topical Thrombin, Gastroenterology 12: 988, 1949.

---

*M/7 phosphate buffer is prepared as follows:
1. Dissolve 20.4 Gm. of disodium phosphate in 1 liter of water.
2. Dissolve 1.95 Gm. of potassium dihydrogenphosphate in 100 c.c. of water.
3. Mix the two solutions.

CHAPTER III

GENITOURINARY EMERGENCIES

ANURIA

A sudden reduction in the amount of urinary excretion calls for immediate consideration of its cause.

A. A palpable bladder suggests obstruction somewhere along the urethra or at the neck of the bladder. In cases of ulceration or inflammation of the external meatus, warm compresses or hot baths may be helpful for temporary relief. If these measures do not relieve the obstruction, the meatus may be gently spread apart and/or a small filiform bougie may be introduced a few centimeters into the urethra in order to facilitate the passage of urine. Sometimes following these procedures the patient still cannot urinate because of sphincter spasm. In some instances prompt relief is afforded by pouring warm water over the external genitals. If all these measures fail it is absolutely necessary to pass a small catheter into the bladder, using sterile conditions. The permanent alleviation of the obstruction in most cases will eventually be a surgical problem.

B. When the bladder is not felt, the etiology of anuria or oliguria may be:

1. Outside the kidney; i.e., cardiac decompensation or dehydration.
2. A disease of the kidney itself.
   (a) In acute glomerulonephritis, in addition to supportive treatment one may either withhold fluids or encourage large amounts orally. In the presence of edema a diuresis may occur with either procedure. If intravenous fluids are required it is best to use a 10% solution of glucose in distilled water, giving 90 c.c. per pound of body weight per twenty-four hours.

ANURIA—Cont'd

B. Nonpalpable bladder—Cont'd

2. A disease of the kidney itself—Cont'd

(b) In chronic glomerulonephritis, the state of uremia and hypertension calls for immediate treatment.

(1) After a blood CO_2 combining power and urea nitrogen are determined, acidosis, if present, should be treated with M/6 sodium lactate solution given intravenously or by clysis as outlined in the section on Diarrhea* (page 27). The desired amount to be given is determined by the following formula:

Normal CO_2 (55) − actual CO_2 × weight in in pounds = total amount of diluted solution to be used.

If the CO_2 is below 20, a 3.75% solution of sodium bicarbonate may be given intravenously. The dosage here is calculated on the assumption that 1 Gm. of sodium bicarbonate per kilogram of body weight will increase the CO_2 by 38 volumes %.

(2) Magnesium sulfate in the following dosage is used if convulsions occur:

Intramuscularly. 50% solution, 0.2 c.c. per kilogram of body weight.

Intravenously. 1% solution, 100-200 c.c. slowly.

Orally, or by rectum. 50% solution, 60-90 c.c.

(3) Calcium gluconate, 5 to 10 c.c. of a 10% solution (diluted 5 times with distilled water), should be given intravenously if there are signs of tetany or extreme depression from the use of magnesium sulfate. (Also see addendum, page 237.)

---

*Whenever alkali is administered to correct acidosis in the presence of renal insufficiency, calcium gluconate should be administered intravenously as indicated on page 53 to prevent the development of convulsions.

ANURIA—Cont'd

B. Nonpalpable bladder—Cont'd

2. A disease of the kidney itself—Cont'd

(b) Chronic glomerulonephritis—treatment of uremia and hypertension —Cont'd

(4) 10% glucose in distilled water may be given if intravenous fluids are required, in amounts of 60-90 c.c. per pound per 24 hours.

(5) Avoid the use of mercurial diuretics.

C. Anuria due to sulfonamide toxicity.

1. Discontinue the drug immediately.
2. Give large amounts of fluids intravenously, 90 to 100 c.c. per pound of body weight per 24 hours, depending on the age and weight of the child.
3. Alkali, M/6 sodium lactate may be used in amounts of 250 to 1000 c.c., depending on the size of the child. (Sodium bicarbonate, 2 gr. per pound per 24 hours, may be given orally if alkali is not given intravenously).

D. Uremia following reaction to blood transfusion (See section on Transfusion Reactions, page 178 et seq.).

GENITOURINARY INJURIES

A. **Conservative Management**

This is indicated whenever shock is mild or disappears promptly and whenever hematuria is not severe or prolonged.

1. Treat shock with plasma or blood.
2. Insure general body rest.
3. Urge large fluid intake.
4. Examine patient periodically.

B. **Surgical Treatment**

This is indicated if hemorrhage is severe or if hematuria and/or anuria persist over 24 hours.

ACUTE RENAL COLIC (URINARY CALCULI)

When the diagnosis is definitely established, morphine (or any of the newer analgesics, such as Demerol, Metopon, or Methadon) should be administered to relieve pain until removal of the calculus is effected. Codeine is rarely of value.

FOREIGN BODY IN GENITOURINARY TRACT

A. **Manual Removal**[1]

Small objects can occasionally be "milked" through urethra to meatus and grasped.

B. **Mechanical Removal**

Urethroscopic or cystoscopic removal is indicated whenever manual removal is not feasible.

ANURIA DUE TO URINARY BLADDER INERTIA RESULTING FROM CENTRAL NERVOUS SYSTEM DISEASE OR INJURY (e.g., Poliomyelitis)

A. Warm applications and gentle pressure to suprapubic area may be useful.

B. Parasympathetic stimulation with various parasympathicomimetic drugs is needed frequently. Among these, Furmethide is very useful in the following doses:[2]

Dosage of Furmethide

AGE OF PATIENT	SUBCUTANEOUS DOSE	ORAL DOSE
0-4 years	1.25-2.5 mg.	2.5 mg. tid.
5-9 years	2.00-3.00 mg.	5.0 mg. tid.
10-19 years	2.50-5.00 mg.	5.0-20.0 mg. tid.
Over 20 years	5.00-7.00 mg.	5.0-20.0 mg. tid.

References

1. Campbell, M. F.: Pediatric Urology, vol. 2, New York, 1937, The Macmillan Co., p. 251.
2. Lawson, R. B.: Therapeutic Problems Encountered in Poliomyelitis, Minnesota Med. 32: 695, 1949.

CHAPTER IV

NEUROLOGICAL EMERGENCIES

CONVULSIONS

Initial treatment is directed at control of the muscular spasm in the safest effective manner. Regardless of cause, persisting convulsions must be rapidly arrested; if uncontrolled, death may occur from exhaustion, hyperthermia, and increased cerebrospinal pressure. All convulsions require sedative therapy. With brief seizures, mild sedation is indicated after the paroxysm to diminish predisposition to further episodes.

A. **Sedation**

1. *Barbiturates.*—The group of choice.

(a) Phenobarbital—The drug of choice.
Dose: 5 to 7 mg. per kilogram of body weight.
Route of administration:

(1) *Intramuscularly.* The dose should vary within the above limits according to the severity and persistence of the seizure. It may be repeated at 20- to 30-minute intervals if convulsions are not controlled.

(2) Rectal sodium phenobarbital may be given in a small retention enema if materials for parenteral injection are not available.

(3) *Orally.* A maintenance dose should be given every 4 to 6 hours after termination of seizure. Elixir phenobarbital may be given in doses of drams 1 to 2 (15 to 30 mg.).

For persisting convulsions or status epilepticus, the following may prove valuable:

(1) The intramuscular administration may be used as outlined above. It will usually prove effective.

CONVULSIONS—Cont'd

A. Sedation—Cont'd

1. *Barbiturates*—Cont'd

(a) Phenobarbital—Cont'd

Persisting convulsions or status epilepticus—Cont'd

(2) Intravenous route—This is most rapidly effective but potentially the most dangerous; *THUS, IT MUST BE USED WITH EXTREME CAUTION.* Rapid administration may precipitate shock; overdose, on the other hand, may precipitate respiratory depression.

Method of administration:

Prepare a 2.5% solution by dissolving 240 mg. of sodium phenobarbital in slightly less than 10 c.c. of isotonic saline or distilled water. Inject 1 c.c. per minute intravenously of this solution slowly and observe the patient closely. When the intensity of the clonic spasm is seen to be diminishing, stop the injection—leave the needle in the vein and observe the patient further. Resume the injection if twitching continues; discontinue when spasms are definitely subsiding.

(b) A variety of other barbiturates may be used.

(1) Nembutal in the form of suppositories (6 mg. or 1/10 gr. per pound—not over 0.4 Gm. or 6 gr. total) may be of value.

(2) Seconal may be administered in the same dose and by the same route.

(3) Pentothal sodium may also be used *rectally;* 0.2 c.c. of a 10% solution per pound of body weight should be injected into the rectum slowly and the patient observed carefully.

2. *Avertin* (Tribromethanol).—For persisting convulsions.

(a) Dosage: 75 mg. per kilogram of body weight administered rectally.

CONVULSIONS—Cont'd

A. Sedation—Cont'd

2. *Avertin*—Cont'd

(b) Method of preparation of Avertin solution:
The calculated dose of avertin in amylene hydrate is dissolved in approximately 40 volumes of distilled water or physiological sodium chloride solution previously heated to exactly 40° C. The solution is shaken vigorously until all globules of Avertin liquid have disappeared. Above 40° C., hydrobromic acid and dibromacetaldehyde may be liberated, and these compounds can cause severe injury to the mucous membranes. The Avertin with amylene hydrate should go completely into solution. If crystals of Avertin appear, the solution must be discarded. Congo red solution is supplied with each bottle of Avertin and is used to test the pH of the mixture. If the Avertin solution is too acid, the Congo red will change to blue or violet. Should this occur, the Avertin must not be used because it is decomposed and, hence, dangerous. The anesthetic solution is used before cooling occurs. Details must be rigidly observed, for improper technique may result in severe reactions, such as hemorrhagic proctitis. Diseases of the rectum and sigmoid contraindicate the use of Avertin.

(c) Method of administration:
Pour 2 to 3 c.c. of the Avertin solution into a funnel attached to the rectal tube. When this amount has been administered, observe the child for several minutes; he may be hypersensitive to Avertin. If the convulsions continue, add another 2 or 3 c.c. of the solution. Continue until convulsions cease or until the calculated amount has been administered. The effect will usually be apparent in 20-30 minutes.

CONVULSIONS—Cont'd
A. Sedation—Cont'd

3. *Magnesium sulfate.*

If there is an antecedent history that would lead one to believe that the convulsions are probably uremic in origin, or if hypertension exists, magnesium sulfate may be given intramuscularly. This is given in a 50% solution. The dose is 0.2 c.c. per kilogram of body weight. This may be repeated every 4-6 hours if necessary. It may also be given intravenously as 100-200 c.c. of a 1% solution, but this must be done very carefully. During intravenous administration the blood pressure should be determined frequently. A 10% solution of calcium gluconate (or chloride) must be available for intravenous use if necessary to counteract any toxic effect of magnesium.

4. *Open drop ether.*

May be used to control convulsions if other drugs are not available or if other methods fail.

B. **Supportive Measures**

1. *General measures.*

The patient must be attended at all times during the seizure and protected with:

(a) Mouth gag to prevent injury to mucous membranes and to provide a patent airway. A rubber or metal airway may be necessary.
(b) Suctioning of secretions to maintain the airway as necessary.
(c) Restraints or padding to prevent injury.

2. *Antipyretic measures.*

Convulsions accompanying fever require sedative therapy as outlined above. Antipyretic measures are used as an adjunct in the general support of the patient.

(a) A cold water enema should be given and may be repeated in 30 to 60 minutes.

CONVULSIONS—Cont'd
B. Supportive Measures—Cont'd
2. *Antipyretic measures*—Cont'd

(b) Tepid sponges: repeated frequently while temperature remains elevated.
(c) Antipyretic medication:
Aspirin—1 gr. per year of age up to 5 years.*
5 gr. for children over 5 years.
Repeat in ½ hour and every 4 hours for the first 24 hours if necessary. The aspirin may be given orally or as a retention enema.

3. *Oxygen.*
Oxygen in high concentration whether given by oxygen tent or mask is a very useful adjunct for reducing intracranial pressure. The value of oxygen is especially marked in prolonged convulsions. If a tent is used, flood the tent with 100% oxygen and then allow the oxygen to flow in at 8-10 liters per minute.

4. *Lumbar puncture.*
Lumbar puncture is necessary at times to relieve pressure as well as to aid in diagnosis. There may be, however, a great degree of danger involved in this procedure. *One preliminary measure that should be observed is a careful examination of the eye grounds to attempt to rule out markedly increased intracranial pressure. This is especially true in cases of specific focal lesions.*

C. **Emergency Diagnostic Measures to Determine Etiology of Convulsions**

1. Blood chemistry.
   (a) N.P.N.
   (b) Calcium.
   (c) Sugar.
2. Spinal fluid examination as directed under section on Meningitis (page 57).
3. Blood culture.

---

*Aspirin should be used with extreme caution in the newborn or young infant because poor renal excretory mechanisms for the salicyl radical may lead to toxicity.

D. Special Considerations

1. *Alkalosis.*

Alkalosis is a relatively uncommon cause of convulsions in infants and children; however, it may be caused by excessive administration of alkali, by excessive loss of chloride resulting from persistent vomiting, or by hyperventilation.

Treatment.

(a) A blood sample for CO_2 combining power and/or blood pH is essential to aid in therapy.
(b) Start an intravenous transfusion of 5% glucose in normal saline. Depending on the severity of dehydration, use from 150 to 300 c.c. of fluid per kilogram of body weight in the first 24 hours.
(c) Subsequent therapy should be adjusted to maintain fluid and electrolyte equilibrium.

Occasionally, severe metabolic or respiratory alkalosis may require more vigorous therapy.

Metabolic Alkalosis.

(a) Intravenous administration of 0.75 c.c. of concentrated hydrochloric acid added to 1 liter of Ringer's solution—slowly.
(b) 30% CO_2 with 70% oxygen should be used followed by 5% CO_2 with 95% oxygen.
(c) Calcium chloride should be administered intravenously. 0.25 to 0.50 c.c. per kilogram of a 5% solution of calcium chloride diluted with equal quantities of distilled water may be administered slowly.
(d) 60 c.c. per kilogram of a mixture of equal parts of M/6 ammonium chloride and Ringer's solution, subcutaneously, may be a more effective method.

Respiratory Alkalosis

(a) Oxygen with CO_2 is usually sufficient.

CONVULSIONS—Cont'd
D. Special Considerations—Cont'd

2. *Hypoglycemia.*

It must be remembered that hypoglycemia may be the cause of convulsions and coma in persons without diabetes as well as in those with diabetes (insulin overdosage). This should be considered despite the absence of a history of diabetes. If the blood sugar level is below 30 mg. %, the patient is usually in severe shock. Early symptoms are sudden hunger, weakness, restlessness, nervousness, pallor or flushing, dilated pupils, and increased pulse rate. Glucose orally or intravenously is necessary to alleviate the symptoms.

(I) *Mild cases* (not accompanied by unconsciousness).

(a) In absence of vomiting:
Orange juice, milk, crackers are usually sufficient.

(b) In presence of vomiting:
(1) When urine contains some sugar, infuse 500-1000 c.c. of 5% glucose in water.
(2) When urine is sugar free, use 20-50 c.c. of 50% glucose in addition to above.

(II) *Severe cases* (associated with partial or complete unconsciousness).

(a) 5-10% glucose in water should be given until urine contains sugar. Clinical signs of improvement appear very slowly in these cases.
(b) Epinephrin (1:1000), ½ minim per kilogram of body weight, is only useful and indicated if regular insulin was being used.
(c) Do not give insulin even though ketones appear in the urine. These may be due to starvation ketosis.

3. *Tetanus.*

The severity of the convulsions in tetanus usually requires vigorous sedation. Not infrequently the judi-

CONVULSIONS—Cont'd
D. Special Considerations—Cont'd
Tetanus—Cont'd

cious combination of several common sedatives and antispasmodic agents offers optimum relaxation. The use of curare has been recently advocated: its exact value is not completely established, however. Nevertheless, its use will be discussed below.

The various agents listed below may be used alone or in combination in accordance with the response of the patient. In general, the optimum and safe dosage of each agent must be determined in each individual case. It must be emphasized, however, that frequently all sedatives have a respiratory depressant action in high concentration.

(a) *Barbiturates.*

(1) As outlined in general section on Convulsions (page 41).

(2) Intravenous Pentothal Sodium in fractional doses under the supervision of an anesthetist may be of distinct value. Although the exact dose necessary to control severe spasms is not definite, good results have been obtained with intravenous doses of 1 to 5 c.c. of a 2% or 2.5% solution. (For a detailed discussion of this method and its merits, refer to the original article.[1])

(b) *Chloral hydrate.*

0.4 gr. per pound of body weight (not over 30 gr. total) may be administered rectally in 15 c.c. of olive oil or 8 c.c. of water.

(c) *Curare.*

A test dose of 0.50 to 0.75 c.c. of aqueous curare (Intocostrin, Squibb) is suggested to be given slowly intravenously over a 2-minute period.* The

---

*Before using curare or any of its derivatives the physician should become familiar with its pharmacology and toxicology. In addition, see section on Curare Poisoning and Its Treatment, page 139.

maximum tolerance of the individual is indicated by the development of roving eyes and nystagmus within the 2-minute period.

(1) The initial dose (following the test dose) may generally be 1.0 c.c. of the aqueous curare (Intocostrin, Squibb) intramuscularly (20 units equal 1.0 c.c.).

(2) Subsequent doses may generally be 1.0 c.c. of the crystalline d-Tubocurarine Chloride in wax and oil (Squibb) (30 mg. or 175 units equal 1.0 c.c.) given intramuscularly.

Treatment should be continued as long as spasticity is present (unless signs of toxicity* to curare develop).

(d) *Ether.*

May also be used as mentioned in general section on Convulsions (page 44).

(e) *Supportive therapy.*

It is worthy of note that this phase of treatment is most important from the initial day of treatment.

(1) Keep patient quiet in a dark room.

(2) Maintain patent airway:
Suction frequently.
Perform tracheotomy, if necessary.
If tracheotomy is performed, aspirate frequently through tracheotomy tube.

(3) Maintain adequate nutrition by means of judicious use of dextrose, saline, protein hydrolysates, transfusions of plasma or whole blood, and parenteral vitamins.

---

*It is important to recall that evidence has been accumulated to indicate that curare, when given repeatedly, may have accumulative action over a period of days. For this reason, Prostigmine Methylsulfate should always be available for intravenous use as an antidote. An individual well trained in the administration of artificial respiration to children should be available.

CONVULSIONS—Cont'd

D. Special Considerations—Cont'd

3. *Tetanus*—Cont'd

(e) *Supportive therapy*—Cont'd

(4) Prevent secondary infections:
Sulfonamides, 1 to 1½ gr. per pound per day.
Penicillin, at least 1 to 2 million units daily.
Other antibiotic agents as needed.

(5) Maintain adequate oxygen supply.
Oxygen tent.
Positive pressure oxygen.

(6) Catheterize patient as needed.

(7) Hot packs may also be useful in relaxing spastic muscles.

(f) *Antitoxin for treatment of tetanus.*

(1) Tetanus antitoxin (or any other horse serum antitoxin) should never be administered unless the routine given in Table III is closely followed with reference to the determination of sensitivity of the patient.

The following outline should be helpful in avoiding mild to fatal reactions to prophylactic and therapeutic doses of antitetanic serum:

1. Administer tetanus antitoxin only if essential.
   (a) Are the indications present? Can care of the local lesion by itself be adequate?
   (b) Can tetanus toxoid be used in place of tetanus antitoxin? A booster dose of 0.1 c.c. of either fluid or alum-precipitated toxoid is adequate even though tetanus toxoid was injected 5 to 6 years previously. In certain instances (delay, strong local lesions, hemorrhage) a booster dose of tetanus toxoid should be supplemented with 10,000 units of tetanus antitoxin.
2. Determine whether the patient is sensitive to horse serum (history, physical examination, skin tests—already presented in the preceding paragraphs).
3. Under all circumstances, adopt the following measures to avoid reactions to tetanus antitoxin:
   (a) Administer an appropriate antihistamine compound, in sufficient quantity, orally or parenterally (when feasible), at least 30 minutes before

CONVULSIONS—Cont'd

D. Special Considerations—Cont'd

3. *Tetanus*—Cont'd

(f) *Antitoxin for treatment of tetanus*—Cont'd

injecting tetanus antitoxin (no matter what the history, physical examination, or tests reveal).

(b) A syringe containing 2 c.c. of epinephrine hydrochloride (1:1,000) should be immediately available to treat any acute serum reactions.

(c) A syringe containing 5 c.c. of diphenhydramine hydrochloride (for intravenous injection) should be immediately available to assist in the control of acute serum actions (1 to 2 c.c. to be injected, and repeated as necessary).

TABLE III. CUTANEOUS TESTS

(From Queries and Minor Notes: J. A. M. A., 1949.[2])

TECHNIQUE	REMARKS
A. Scratch test 1. Make 2 superficial scratches on front (volar) surface of either forearm 2. Apply a drop of 1:10 dilution (0.1 c.c. serum in 9.9 c.c. of isotonic NaCl solution) over upper scratch (use lower scratch as control) 3. If, after 15 to 20 minutes, no local or constitutional reaction occurs, proceed to the intracutaneous test, described under 4 B. Intracutaneous test 4. Raise a tiny wheal (smallest amount of serum practicable) on the front (volar) aspect of either forearm 5. Use the following dilutions: Presumptive positive sensitivity:* 1:10,000 dilution; negative sensitivity:* 1:1,000 dilution Under all circumstances: at 15- to 20-minute intervals, if preceding dilutions give negative readings, repeat tests in the order of the next lower dilution: 1:1,000, 1:100, 1:10	1. Positive local reaction: area of edema about 0.5 inch in diameter with erythema (like a wheal), with or without finger-like projections at circumference (pseudopodia), appears within 15 to 20 minutes 2. A negative reaction does not always mean that it is safe to give serum 3. A positive reaction does not always indicate that it is dangerous to give serum 4. But, when a positive reaction does prove to indicate clinical sensitivity, the sooner the reaction, and the greater its size, the greater is the likelihood of a constitutional (anaphylactic reaction 5. The tests must be given each time serum is to be injected (may change from positive to negative or vice versa) 6. Constitutional reactions (various forms of "serum sickness") to skin tests are identical with those which follow injections of serum for prophylaxis or therapy; they may follow with either negative or positive skin reactions

*Presumptive diagnosis of serum sensitivity: (a) presence of allergic complaints (hay fever, asthma, hives, food sensitivities, migraine, eczema, etc.) in the patient or relatives (past or present); (b) serum injections in the past (tetanus, diphtheria, pneumonia, etc.) without any reaction (early or late). Probable sensitivity: (a) skin reactions (or ophthalmic reactions) positive on previous occasions; (b) allergic complaints (sneezing, coughing, wheezing, burning eyes, stomach ache, hives, itching, headache, etc.) when around horses (if horse serum is to be used) or cows (if bovine serum is to be used). Positive sensitivity: (a) allergic difficulties from previous injections of horse serum; (b) constitutional (anaphylactic) reactions from cutaneous or ophthalmic tests for sensitivity; (c) constitutional reaction during present injections.

CONVULSIONS—Cont'd

D. Special Considerations—Cont'd

3. *Tetanus*—Cont'd

(f) *Antitoxin for treatment of tetanus*—Cont'd

(d) In the presence of a probable or positive diagnosis of serum sensitivity, the patient should be hospitalized for at least 24 to 48 hours.

(e) All patients who receive tetanus antitoxin (independent of history, physical examination, or tests) should be given one of the antihistamine compounds for fourteen days to avoid all forms of serum sickness. Observe for side effects of antihistaminics.

(f) In the presence of presumptive, probable, or positive diagnosis of serum sensitivity, in addition to antihistamine therapy, hospitalization, and epinephrine hydrochloride (as needed), employ the method of hyposensitization given in Table IV.

(g) At an appropriate interval after serum prophylaxis (4 to 6 weeks after the now recommended dose of 5,000 to 10,000 units) inject 0.5 c.c. of alum-precipitated tetanus toxoid (use the newly marketed purified products) and repeat dose in one month. Thus, on subsequent occasions, tetanus toxoid may be employed in the form of booster doses in place of antitetanic serum.

TABLE IV

DILUTION OF ANTITOXIN	VOLUME	ROUTE	INTERVAL AND REMARKS
1:1,000	0.1 0.2 0.3 0.5 1.0	Subcutaneous	15 minutes between each injection of antitoxin
1:100	0.1 0.2 0.5 1.0	Subcutaneous	In case of reactions during course of injections, treat reactions, continue dose preceding reaction, gradually increase dose if further difficulty is not encountered
1:10	0.1 0.2 0.5 1.0	Subcutaneous	In case of reactions, increase intervals between injections to 30 minutes
None (undiluted)	0.1 0.2 0.5 1.0	Subcutaneous	
	Rest of serum as one dose intramuscularly		

(2) Never use antitoxin that has been frozen.

(3) Warm antitoxin to body temperature before using.

CONVULSIONS—Cont'd

D. Special Considerations—Cont'd

3. *Tetanus*—Cont'd

(f) *Antitoxin for treatment of tetanus*—Cont'd

(4) On admission, 25,000 units of antitoxin should be given intramuscularly. Repeat this dose in 12 hours. Then, 15,000 units of antitoxin intramuscularly should be given each day for 3 to 5 days.

(5) THE INTRAVENOUS METHOD IS NOT DESIRABLE FOR ANY CHILD.

4. *Tetany.*[3]

If the diagnosis of tetany is made clinically, calcium gluconate is the drug of choice; 0.3-1.0 Gm. may be given intravenously in a 2% solution (diluting the 10% solution 5 times). This should be injected slowly and discontinued when the spasms are subsiding. For sustained treatment, 1-2 Gm. of calcium chloride diluted with saline or the child's formula to a 2% solution may be given orally. More concentrated solutions may damage the gastric mucosa.

HEAD INJURY*

1. A complete history should be elicited while the examination is being done. Ascertain whether the patient was unconscious and whether unconsciousness was interrupted by a lucid period; whether unconsciousness was immediate or delayed. A lucid period followed by unconsciousness usually indicates intracranial hemorrhage, and, therefore, generally requires surgical intervention.
2. If convulsions are present, a record should be kept with reference to their character and distribution.
3. The eyes should be carefully examined:
   (a) Eyeball activity may be especially important—presence of roving or nystagmus should be noted.
   (b) Ecchymosis of eyeball.

---

*An additional section is presented in the addendum, page 226.

HEAD INJURY—Cont'd
3. Examination of eyes—Cont'd

(c) Pupil size, equality, and reaction to light.
(d) Appearance of fundus—with special reference to retinal hemorrhage.

4. The scalp should be examined for external injury and for any depressions before either edema or hematoma forms.
5. Examination of the ears, nose, and mouth should be done in order to note any bleeding or cerebrospinal leakage. Later, the mastoid regions, the eyes, and the neck should be observed for the presence of ecchymosis; this may be an indication of the site of the fracture.
6. The reflexes are to be examined and recorded.
7. The temperature should be taken every half hour.
8. The pulse and respirations should be taken every 15 minutes. A slow pulse, deepening coma, slow respiratory rate, and noisy respirations are indicative of increasing intracranial pressure.
9. The blood pressure should be taken every 6 hours.
10. The urine should be examined (catheterize, if necessary.
11. Spinal tap as a routine measure is not advisable, except in the presence of definite signs of increased intracranial pressure. If a spinal tap is performed, the fluid should be collected in three different tubes. The presence of blood in all three tubes is evidence of bleeding. If blood is found in only one tube and a slight amount in the second tube, the bleeding is the result of a traumatic lumbar puncture.

Initial Treatment

1. Oxygen inhalation is essential in the treatment of shock, particularly if the persistent coma is on the basis of cerebral edema; the administration of oxygen may shorten the comatose period considerably.

HEAD INJURY—Cont'd
Initial Treatment—Cont'd

2. Infusion of plasma or whole blood in cases accompanied by blood loss.
3. If available, the intravenous administration of 25 c.c. of concentrated human serum albumin may be of value in reducing cerebral edema. Magnesium sulfate may also be used as outlined in the section on Convulsions (page 44).
4. Keep the patient warm.
5. Do not give morphine sulfate or codeine. Barbiturates may be used cautiously for sedation, if necessary.
6. Apply ice cap.
7. Keep the patient quiet, flat, and avoid excitement.
8. Protect all wounds with sterile dressings. Carefully cleanse the scalp about the wound with warm water and soap. Shave and cleanse the surrounding area with ether and alcohol; paint with tincture of iodine, followed with alcohol to prevent burning tender skin.
9. Examine the depth of the wound; not any fractures.
10. When there is bleeding or drainage from the ears or nose, cleanse the surrounding areas and apply a loose sterile dressing so as to allow for free drainage; *do not pack.* Free drainage is essential.
11. When there is bleeding from the nose, mouth, or ears, or drainage of cerebrospinal fluid, place the patient in a position to allow for free drainage. There is no objection to placing the patient on his side or abdomen, or elevating the patient's head to afford better drainage if it is not contraindicated by complicating fracture.
12. Maintain free airway. Suction whenever necessary.
13. Catheterize as often as needed to relieve bladder distention.
14. X-ray the patient only when he has recovered from shock. Negative x-ray does not preclude the presence

HEAD INJURY—Cont'd
Initial Treatment—Cont'd
14. X-raying—Cont'd

of a fracture. A fracture of the skull in itself is not of serious nature; the danger occurs only when there is damage to the intracranial contents.

A child reacts readily from head injury, and as soon as he does he may be allowed to move about. Tying children down in bed and making them fight against restraint is not good practice. The child should be kept in bed for two days after symptoms have disappeared. Neurosurgical consultation is essential.

COMA

Coma is only a sign of underlying disease or injury. The determination of its etiology is of primary importance, since the treatment depends almost entirely upon the cause. The more common causes of coma are:

Head injury
Meningitis (all types)
Acute encephalitis
Uremia
Diabetes and hypoglycemia
Acute infectious diseases
Poisons
Intracranial hemorrhage in the newborn
Brain tumor

Less common causes include:

Subdural hematoma
Extradural hematoma
Epilepsy
Cerebral embolism, cerebral thrombosis, hepatic insufficiency, burns, drowning, and hysteria

COMA—Cont'd

HEAD INJURY

(See Section on Head Injury, page 53)

MENINGITIS

The diagnosis of meningitis may frequently be a difficult one to make clinically, especially in the young infant or child. If meningitis is suspected, therefore, the following procedures and treatment should be instituted as soon as possible:

A. *SPINAL TAP.* Obtain pressure readings, if possible. Collect 3 specimens of fluid.
   1. Routine spinal fluid examination should include:
      (a) Physical appearance.
      (b) Cell count and differential.
      (c) Direct smear of concentrated specimen for organisms—Gram stain.
      (d) Use of the various specific diagnostic sera for organism as seen on smear.
      (e) Culture for predominating organism including special culture methods for *Hemophilus influenzae* and *Mycobacterium tuberculosis.* If organism is obtained on culture, the sensitivity of the organism to the sulfonamides and *all* available antibiotics should be determined as rapidly as possible.
      (f) If tuberculosis is suspected, inoculate a guinea pig by appropriate technique.
      (g) Chemistry: (1) sugar, (2) protein, (3) chlorides.

B. If spinal fluid is cloudy or purulent in appearance, inject intrathecally
   1. 10,000 units of penicillin
   2. 25 to 50 mg. of streptomycin diluted in about 5 c.c. of physiological saline.

C. Obtain a complete blood count, blood culture, hematocrit, and CO_2 combining power.

D. Start continuous intravenous fluid administration; perform a "cut down" on an appropriate vein if necessary.

COMA—Cont'd
Meningitis—Cont'd

E. Administer aqueous adrenal cortical extract intravenously (as outlined in the section on Acute Adrenal Insufficiency, page 67) if the child is very toxic or shows signs of collapse.

F. Institute combined chemotherapy and antibiotic therapy because:
   1. Causative organism may not be known for a variable period.
   2. Vigorous treatment is necessary and imperative in most forms of meningitis. The mortality rate for meningitis is still *too* high. In addition, neurological sequelae are still too frequent in those who are tided over the acute phase.
      (a) *Sulfadiazine.**
         (1) Of prime importance before administering sulfadiazine is the establishment and maintenance of adequate urine output. Adequate hydration of the patient is obtained by the use of 5% glucose in water alternated with 5% glucose in saline intravenously. If the CO_2 combining power is low, it is necessary first to correct the condition by the administration of alkali in sufficient doses as outlined in section on Diarrhea (page 27). Infants should receive on the average of 3 ounces of fluid per pound of body weight in the first 24 hours. If dehydration is very severe, they may require up to 4 or 5 ounces per pound of body weight in the first 24 hours. It is imperative to correct the fluid balance before transfusion is given. During the sulfonamide administration 40 c.c. of molar lactate added to each 1000 c.c. of fluid may generally be expected to prevent crystalluria.

*Use of combined sulfonamide therapy may further reduce toxicity of individual sulfonamides. For parenteral use, sulfadiazine-sulfamerazine combined (equal amounts of each to provide total dosage as indicated on page 59) is probably best.

COMA—Cont'd
MENINGITIS—Cont'd
F. Combined chemotherapy and antibiotic therapy—Cont'd
2. Treatment—Cont'd
(a) *Sulfadiazine*—Cont'd

(2) *Dosage of sulfadiazine:* 1½ to 2 gr. per pound of body weight per 24 hours should be given in divided doses as indicated below.

(3) *Method of administration:*

Subcutaneously. Sodium sulfadiazine may be used as either an 0.5% or a 5% solution. One-half of the total daily dosage should be given every 12 hours. It is usually advisable to continue this route of administration until the patient is able to take medication by mouth. However, if continued orally, careful check of blood levels should be made regularly to ensure an adequate therapeutic level.

Intravenously. The intravenous route of administration may also be used after hydration has been established. (This method, however, may prove to be somewhat more hazardous than the subcutaneous route because of the establishment of very high peak levels). One-half of the total daily dosage may be given initially and the remainder may be given in equally divided doses every 4 hours.* A 5% solution of sodium sulfadiazine should be used. It may be easily prepared by dissolving 5 Gm. of the sterile powder of sodium sulfadiazine (using sterile precautions) in 100 c.c. of sterile distilled water, or by the addition of 45 c.c. of sterile distilled water to an ampule containing 2.5 Gm. of the sodium sulfadiazine in 5 c.c. of solution. Each cubic centimeter of the prepared solution will contain 0.75 gr.

*An alternate method is the use of continuous intravenous drip in which the total amount is administered over a 24-hour period.

COMA—Cont'd

MENINGITIS—Cont'd

F. Combined chemotherapy and antibiotic therapy—Cont'd

2. Treatment—Cont'd

(a) *Sulfadiazine*—Cont'd

(3) *Method of administration*—Cont'd

Intravenously—Cont'd

(0.05 Gm.) of sodium sulfadiazine. Thus, one may easily calculate the required number of cubic centimeters of prepared solution to be given at each time. Generally, the intravenous method is continued until the patient is able to take medication by mouth.

(b) *Penicillin.*

In addition to the initial intrathecal dose, 100,000 units of crystalline penicillin G in isotonic saline should be administered intramuscularly or intravenously every 2 hours. The initial dose should be given intravenously.

(c) *Streptomycin.*

In addition to the initial intrathecal dose, 20 mg. per pound per day of dihydrostreptomycin should be administered either intramuscularly or subcutaneously in 4 equally divided doses.

(d) *Other antibiotics.*

In the line of recent development it may be of value to add aureomycin, both intravenously and orally. Although optimum doses in the treatment of meningitis remain to be established, high doses (100 to 200 mg.) of *properly buffered* aureomycin have been given intravenously without evidence of toxicity. These high doses have produced adequate spinal fluid levels of aureomycin. Aureomycin should also be given orally in doses of 25 to 50 mg. per kilogram of body weight per 24 hours in divided doses given every 4 hours.

Terramycin—See addendum, page 234.

COMA—Cont'd
MENINGITIS—Cont'd

G. *SPECIFIC THERAPY.*

As soon as the etiologic agent is determined by the bacteriologist, a change in the therapeutic approach should be made according to the following plan.*

1. *PNEUMOCOCCIC MENINGITIS.*

Although penicillin is the most important agent in the treatment of pneumococcic meningitis, combined penicillin and sulfadiazine should be the method of choice.

(a) *Sulfadiazine* should be continued in doses of 1½ to 2 gr. per pound per day, either subcutaneously, orally, or intravenously, in proper dilutions. If given orally, daily blood levels should be taken to make certain that a therapeutic level (approximately 15 mg. %) is maintained.

(b) *Penicillin.*†

(1) Children under 2 years of age should receive 500,000 units of crystalline penicillin G in aqueous solution intramuscularly every 2 hours.

(2) Children over 2 years of age should receive 1,000,000 units of crystalline penicillin G in aqueous solution intramuscularly every 2 hours.

The optimum duration of treatment has still not been established. However, the treatment as outlined above should be continued for at least 14

*Although this plan is presented, it should be considered a flexible one and the treatment should be adapted to each individual case, depending on the needs. One cannot emphasize too strongly that the use of antibiotic agents should not eliminate the real need for careful observation of the patient and his progress not only with reference to the meningitis, but also with reference to the development of secondary complications; for example, pneumonia of various types may be expected to develop because of the immobility of the patient.

†The intrathecal route is no longer recommended by us in the treatment of pneumococcic meningitis, although it is still used in some hospitals. The use of huge doses of penicillin intramuscularly at frequent intervals as suggested in the outline establishes very high spinal fluid penicillin levels, ensures adequate cerebral distribution, and is unassociated with neurotoxicity which sometimes resulted from intrathecal administration of penicillin. In addition, the large doses are well tolerated.

COMA—Cont'd

MENINGITIS—Cont'd

G. *SPECIFIC THERAPY*—Cont'd

1. *PNEUMOCOCCIC MENINGITIS*—Cont'd

(b) *Penicillin*—Cont'd

days after the last sterile spinal fluid culture and after the temperature has become normal. Other antibiotic agents should be added to or substituted for penicillin should drug resistance of the offending organism develop.

2. *H. INFLUENZAE MENINGITIS.*

Combined sulfadiazine, penicillin, streptomycin, and specific rabbit antiserum is the method of choice in the severely ill patient.*

(a) *Sulfadiazine.* Administer as outlined under Pneumococcic Meningitis (page 61).

(b) *Streptomycin.*

Intramuscular administration: 20 mg. per pound per day of dihydrostreptomycin should be continued in 2 to 4 equally divided doses daily for 3 to 4 days.

Intrathecal Administration: 25 to 50 mg. of streptomycin (*not* dihydrostreptomycin) once daily for 2 or 3 days.

(c) *Type-specific rabbit antiserum.*

(1) *Determination of initial dose* (Method of H. Alexander[10]):

SPINAL FLUID SUGAR IN MG. %	DOSE OF TYPE SPECIFIC ANTISERUM IN MG.
15 or less	100
15 to 24	75
25 to 40	50
Over 40	25

*Other antibiotic agents have also been suggested as adjuvant agents in the therapy of this type of meningitis. Sufficient experience has not yet been had to demonstrate their real value or to establish optimum dosage schedules. Penicillin, for example, has been suggested as an adjunct in treatment because some strains of *H. influenzae* are very susceptible to penicillin and also because secondary pyogenic organisms may readily be controlled by penicillin. Aureomycin has recently been suggested in cases of *H. influenzae* meningitis both intravenously and orally because in vitro studies have indicated that this antibiotic may be especially useful in *H. influenzae* infections. Polymyxin B has also been suggested. Nevertheless, because of the nephrotoxicity seen with the latter, it should be used only when other agents have been demonstrated to be ineffective.

COMA—Cont'd
MENINGITIS—Cont'd
G. *SPECIFIC THERAPY*—Cont'd
2. *H. INFLUENZAE MENINGITIS*—Cont'd
(c) *Type-specific rabbit antiserum*—Cont'd

(2) *Method of administration.*
(Sensitivity testing, including intracutaneous and ophthalmic, is essential before administration).

Preparation of serum:
Dilute the necessary amount of serum in a volume of isotonic saline so that the total volume of fluid equals 10 c.c. per kilogram of body weight.
Intravenously. This is the method of choice. The total amount of diluted serum should be administered slowly, 10 to 20 drops per minute. Immediate and/or delayed reactions may occur but are never too serious.
Intramuscularly. This method is used only when there is some difficulty in administering intravenous fluids to the patient. The serum should be administered undiluted.

(3) *Determination of subsequent doses.*
(i) If daily spinal taps are done for the administration of streptomycin intrathecally, or for further diagnostic or therapeutic reasons, spinal fluid sugar examinations should be performed and the method of H. Alexander should again be followed.
(ii) On the other hand, if daily spinal fluid sugar determinations are not possible, the dose should be ascertained by the type-specific capsular swelling of the patient's serum.
If capsular swelling is obtained in a 1:10 dilution of the patient's serum, no more

COMA—Cont'd

MENINGITIS—Cont'd

G. *SPECIFIC THERAPY*—Cont'd

2. *H. INFLUENZAE MENINGITIS*—Cont'd

(c) *Type-specific rabbit antiserum*—Cont'd

(3) *Determination of subsequent doses*—Cont'd

(ii)—Cont'd

antiserum is necessary. If no capsular swelling is observed, the dose of serum given on the previous day is repeated.

(d) Penicillin should be administered in doses of 100,000 units every 3 hours intramuscularly.*

The optimum duration of treatment in *H. influenzae* meningitis also remains to be established. However, the following generalities may be made:

(1) Sulfadiazine and penicillin should be continued for at least 7 days after the last sterile spinal fluid and after temperature has returned to normal.

(2) Streptomycin should be continued intramuscularly for no longer than 4 days.

(3) Type-specific rabbit antiserum should be administered only in accordance with the instructions listed above.

Naturally, if during the course of treatment the patient shows poor response, aureomycin,[4, 4-a] Chloromycetin,[11] and/or polymyxin B[5] should be administered if the organism proves sensitive to any of these antibiotics.†[1]

---

*As indicated in another footnote, penicillin is recommended because in vitro tests have revealed many strains of *H. influenzae* which are sensitive to penicillin.

†As mentioned previously, optimum dosage schedules have not been established. Nevertheless, the following suggestions should aid in therapy:

(a) *Aureomycin* or *Chloromycetin*. The combined intravenous and oral method is probably the method of choice.
  (1) Intravenous—5 mg. per kilogram of properly buffered aureomycin hydrochloride every 6 hours.
  (2) Oral—20 to 50 mg. per kilogram of body weight per day in divided doses given every 4 to 6 hours.

(b) *Polymyxin B*. Extreme caution should be exercised before selecting polymyxin B because of its nephrotoxicity. The combined intramuscular and intrathecal administration is probably necessary.
  (1) Intramuscular—5 mg. per kilogram per day in divided doses given every 4 to 6 hours.
  (2) Intrathecal—1 mg. per day.

COMA—Cont'd
MENINGITIS—Cont'd
G. *SPECIFIC THERAPY*—Cont'd

3. *MENINGOCOCCIC MENINGITIS.*
   (a) Sulfadiazine is the drug of choice—dose as described in section on Pneumococcic Meningitis (page 61).
   (b) Penicillin should be used in addition in severe cases and especially in the presence of either meningococcal conjunctivitis or bacteremia. Treatment should be continued for at least 72 hours after the temperature becomes normal.
4. *TUBERCULOSIS MENINGITIS.*
   Effective therapy depends on early diagnosis. Combined streptomycin and promizole therapy offers the greatest possible chance of cure at present.
   (a) *Streptomycin.* Although optimum doses have not been established, combined intramuscular and intrathecal administration over long periods of time is apparently essential.
      (1) *Intramuscularly.* Dihydrostreptomycin should be administered in doses of 30 mg. per pound per day either in 2 equally divided doses or in one daily dose. This should be continued for approximately 6 months.
      (2) *Intrathecally.* 50 to 100 mg. of streptomycin (*not dihydrostreptomycin*) should be administered daily for approximately 40 days. Should technical difficulties arise, suitable rest periods should be planned during which time no intrathecal medication is administered.
   (b) *Promizole.* Administered orally at 6-hour intervals so that total daily dosage is 1.0 to 8.0 Gm. daily. Dosage is adjusted so that blood level of 2-3 mg. % is attained.

COMA—Cont'd
MENINGITIS—Cont'd
G. *SPECIFIC THERAPY*—Cont'd
4. *TUBERCULOSIS MENINGITIS*—Cont'd
(b) *Promizole*—Cont'd

Para-aminosalicylic acid is also being used in some clinics in doses of 0.2 Gm. per kilogram per day in 4 equally divided doses.

5. *FRIEDLANDER'S BACILLUS MENINGITIS.*
Therapy with sulfadiazine and streptomycin should be instituted as outlined under section on *H. Influenzae* Meningitis (page 62). Aureomycin and Chloromycetin may also be useful.

6. *E. COLI MENINGITIS.*
This type of meningitis is most commonly seen in the newborn period and in early infancy.
(a) Streptomycin should be administered as outlined in section on H. Influenzae Meningitis (page 62).
(b) Aureomycin should be administered in doses of 25 to 50 mg. per kilogram per day in 4 equally divided doses orally for approximately 7 to 10 days. If the patient is critically ill or if the medication is not tolerated orally, the intravenous route, using properly buffered solution which is available commercially, is recommended.
(c) *Chloromycetin* (chloramphenicol) should also be administered orally in doses of 25 to 50 mg. per kilogram per day if the organism proves sensitive.

7. *STAPHYLOCOCCIC MENINGITIS.**
(a) Penicillin and sulfadiazine should be administered as outlined in section on Pneumococcic Meningitis (page 61). Two weeks of such treatment should be the minimum length of time.
(b) Occasionally, streptomycin or aureomycin may be necessary either to supplement penicillin and sulfadiazine or to be used in place of penicillin.†

*For bacitracin therapy, see addendum, page 231.

†It is well to point out that a recent report[7] indicated that aureomycin was more effective in a particular case of staphylococcic meningitis when the penicillin and sulfadiazine were discontinued.

COMA—Cont'd
MENINGITIS—Cont'd
G. *SPECIFIC THERAPY*—Cont'd

8. *MENINGITIS ACCOMPANIED BY BACTEREMIA WITH ACUTE ADRENAL INSUFFICIENCY.*

The association of bacteremia and acute adrenal insufficiency is generally referred to as the Waterhouse-Friderichsen syndrome. It most commonly develops in cases associated with meningococcic infections. However, it may develop during the course of any meningitis and, furthermore, may develop very early in the course of the infectious process when meningeal signs have not yet developed. Early diagnosis is imperative. There may be a preceding upper respiratory infection, but the onset is usually abrupt, with sudden chills, fever, malaise, and early appearance of petechiae and purpuric spots. This is usually followed by cyanosis and collapse. There are two important clinical observations which may be of real value even before petechiae develop. These are a progressive increase in the pulse rate associated with a progressive decrease in blood pressure. Thus, during management frequent blood pressure readings offer an excellent guide as to the progress of the patient.

Treatment.

(a) Take blood for culture, sodium, potassium, chlorides, N.P.N., CO_2 combining power, sugar, and hematocrit determinations, if possible.

(b) Administer aqueous adrenal cortical extract intravenously or intramuscularly in divided doses every 2 hours. The total dose in 24 hours should be equivalent to 2 c.c. per pound. Half of this amount may be given as a stat dose.

(c) If aqueous adrenal cortical extract is not available, desoxycorticosterone acetate in oil (Doca) may be

COMA—Cont'd

MENINGITIS—Cont'd

G. *SPECIFIC THERAPY*—Cont'd

8. *MENINGITIS ACCOMPANIED BY BACTEREMIA WITH ACUTE ADRENAL INSUFFICIENCY*—Cont'd

Treatment—Cont'd

(c) Cont'd

used. However, Doca must be used with caution since overdose may produce hemodilution, edema, hypertension, and cardiac failure. It should be given intramuscularly every 6 or 8 hours for 3 or 4 doses.

PATIENT'S WEIGHT IN KG.	DOSE IN C.C.
5	0.4
10	0.5
20	1.0
30	2.5

(d) Sulfadiazine (sodium) intravenously, as outlined previously. Blood level should be 15 mg. per 100 c.c.

(e) Penicillin as outlined under treatment of Pneumococcic Meningitis (page 61).

(f) Fluids, 5% glucose in saline or Hartmann's solution.
  (1) Immediate dose of 30 c.c. per kilogram of body weight.
  (2) Follow at a rate to give 150 c.c. per kilogram of body weight per day.

(g) Observe blood pressure every 2 hours for first 12 hours.

(h) Large doses of plasma for shock, ephedrine sulfate to elevate blood pressure, and oxygen for cyanosis.

(i) In newborn infants with acute adrenal insufficiency it is important that vitamin K be given intravenously (5-10 mg.) in addition.

ACUTE ENCEPHALITIS

There are many types of encephalitis, the most definite types being as follows:

COMA—Cont'd
ACUTE ENCEPHALITIS—Cont'd

Epidemic encephalitis
Acute polioencephalitis
Encephalitis following vaccination
Encephalitis complicating acute contagious diseases
Encephalitis due to poisoning, such as lead or arsenic
Encephalitis due to toxoplasmosis

Treatment

1. Lumbar puncture; spinal fluid as under routine spinal tap and also spinal fluid sent to virus laboratory.
2. Anticonvulsant (barbiturates, Avertin—as previously described, page 42 et seq.).
3. Hot packs or baths.
4. Parenteral feeding as indicated.
5. Use of antibiotics to prevent secondary infection.
6. General supportive therapy, including oxygen.

UREMIA (See Section on Genitourinary Emergencies, page 37 et seq.)

DIABETES AND HYPOGLYCEMIA

Coma may occur in diabetic children as a result of hypoglycemia or severe ketosis. The term coma, however, in diabetes is generally reserved for the state of unconsciousness due to severe ketosis.

Ketosis in diabetic children develops more rapidly than in diabetic adults because of the small stores of liver glycogen in children, the frequency of acute infections, and the tendency of many parents to withhold insulin in the presence of vomiting or refusal of food.

When an acute infection or other metabolic strain is encountered by the diabetic child, there is an increased need for insulin. If the additional insulin is not made available to the child, the blood sugar begins to rise and liver glycogen decreases. When the blood sugar level rises above the renal

COMA—Cont'd
DIABETES—Cont'd

threshhold, the sugar is excreted into the urine. As the stores of glycogen in the liver decrease, fat is metabolized by the liver in increased quantities, producing large quantities of ketone bodies. When the concentration of ketone bodies in the blood rises above the maximum level for utilization by the muscles, these ketone bodies are excreted in the urine and through the lungs. The patient becomes dehydrated because there is an increased excretion of water in the urine for dissolving the excreted glucose and ketone bodies. Acidosis develops because of the increase in ketone bodies in the blood and the depletion of fixed base of the body when the fixed base is excreted in combination with the ketone bodies in the urine.

Treatment of diabetic coma is aimed at correcting the disturbed carbohydrate metabolism as rapidly as possible. The interplay of several factors makes it impossible to predict with any degree of exactness the amounts of insulin, water, glucose, and alkali that will be required to overcome ketosis in any given case. The use of formulae to calculate the requirements of these elements is, therefore, not indicated. A simple method may be used for all children in diabetic coma, and adjustments may be made for each individual case. The schedule is modeled after that suggested by Hartmann.[8]

Treatment of Diabetic Coma*

1. *Insulin*

   2 units of regular insulin per kilogram of body weight is to be given subcutaneously at once. A second dose of insulin is to be given 6 hours later, between ¼ and 1 unit of regular insulin per kilogram of body weight, the exact amount to vary according to the child's needs.

2. *Water and Alkali*

   30 c.c. M/6 sodium lactate per kilogram of body weight is to be given intravenously in the first 6 hours. Thirty cubic centimeters of M/6 sodium lactate per kilogram

*An alternate plan is presented in the addendum, page 232.

COMA—Cont'd
DIABETES—Cont'd
Treatment of Diabetic Coma—Cont'd
2. *Water and Alkali*—Cont'd

and 40 c.c. of hypotonic Ringer's* solution per kilogram are to be given subcutaneously. If the coma, ketosis, and dehydration have not been overcome after 6 hours, a supplementary injection of M/6 sodium lactate, 30 c.c. per kilogram of body weight, should be given intravenously. Glucose need not be given parenterally because of the glucogenic effects of the sodium lactate which is administered.

3. Gastric aspiration should be done to avoid dilatation of the stomach and vomiting.
4. Since diabetic coma is frequently associated with infection, the symptoms of which may be masked by the coma, it is wise to initiate antibiotic therapy on admission.

TABLE V.

	FIRST 6 HOURS	SECOND 6 HOURS
Insulin	2 units/kilogram	¼ to 1 unit/kilogram
Water	100 c.c./kilogram	30 c.c./kilogram
Alkali (includes water requirement)	30 c.c./kilogram M/6 Na lactate intravenously 30 c.c. per kilogram M/6 Na lactate and 40 c.c./kilogram hypotonic Ringer's solution subcutaneously	30 c.c./kilogram M/6 Na lactate intravenously

Laboratory tests should be done before instituting treatment and during the course of treatment whenever possible. Before instituting treatment, blood should be examined for its CO_2 combining power or CO_2 content, and the concentration of sugar should be determined. Urine should be examined for sugar and ketone bodies (catheterize if necessary). During the course of treatment the urine should be examined for sugar and ketone bodies every 2 hours until these abnormal substances have disappeared. A second blood sugar determination is advisable 6 hours after the institution of treatment. Failure of the patient to respond promptly to

*For composition see Table II, page 30.

COMA—Cont'd
DIABETES—Cont'd
Treatment of Diabetic Coma—Cont'd

these therapeutic measures should lead the physician to search for an undiscovered infection.

The third and fourth 6-hour periods of treatment may be modeled after the second 6-hour period in Table V. Oral feeding may be started when the patient is no longer vomiting and when the patient is clear mentally.

The further treatment may be modeled after the regime of Woodyatt[12] as follows:

> Each day is divided into 4 periods of 6 hours each. At the beginning of each period the urine is tested for sugar and for acetone. If there is sugar or acetone in the urine an injection of regular insulin is given. If the amount of sugar in the urine increases from one period to the next, the amount of insulin to be injected also increases. If the amount of sugar in the urine decreases in subsequent periods, the additional insulin may be reduced in quantity. Insulin dosage may be determined on the basis of the percentage of sugar in the urine, as shown in Table VI.

In each 6-hour period the patient must receive by mouth water and sugar. Fruit juice may usually be relied upon in the early stages to be taken well by mouth and to supply the required quantities of both water and sugar since orange juice may generally be considered to be a 10% solution of glucose. This regime is shown schematically on the opposite page.

After 24 hours or more of the Woodyatt regime if the patient continues to progress satisfactorily as evidenced by alertness, normal respirations, no evidence of acidosis or dehydration and provided fluids are retained by mouth, a soft

TABLE VI. INSULIN NEEDS DURING THERAPY

URINE SUGAR	REGULAR INSULIN
0-2%	5 units
2-4%	10 units
4-6%	15 units
6%+	20 units

COMA—Cont'd
DIABETES—Cont'd
Treatment of Diabetic Coma—Cont'd

Woodyatt Regime

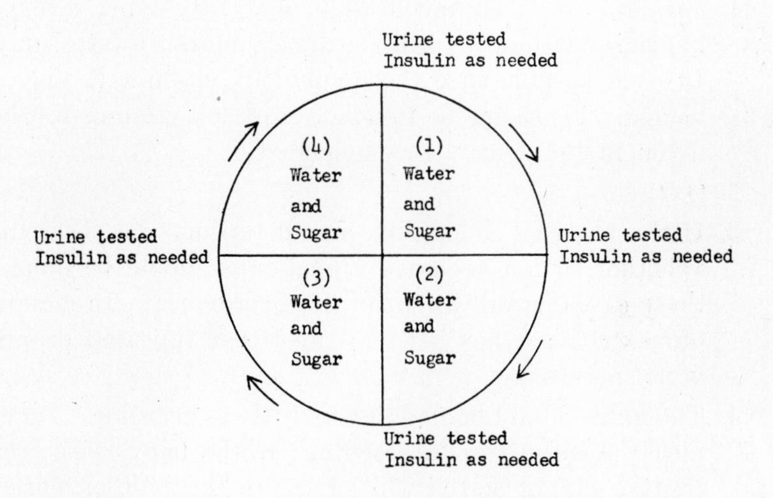

Water requirement	250 to 400 cc in each 6-hour period.
Sugar	25 to 40 Gm. in each 6-hour period.

full caloric diet may be offered, but the urine should be continued to be tested and regular insulin given as indicated in Table VI.

ACUTE INFECTIOUS DISEASES (Such as Brain Abscesses and Cavernous Sinus Thrombosis)

A. In addition to the anticonvulsant therapy, specific chemotherapeutic measures are indicated, as outlined in section on Meningitis (page 57).

B. Oxygen if indicated.

POISONS (See Section on Poisoning, Chapter VII)

COMA—Cont'd

INTRACRANIAL HEMORRHAGE IN THE NEWBORN

Treatment

1. Vitamin K subcutaneously, 5 mg. stat; 1 mg. every 4 hours for 48 hours. 1 mg. every 24 hours for 5 to 7 days. In each specific case the amount of vitamin K may be varied. There are no toxic effects from vitamin K when given in the dosage recommended.
2. Oxygen.
3. If the fontanel is bulging, spinal tap may be necessary. Whether or not repeated spinal taps should be done in these cases is still a matter of controversy. In general, our experience has led us to feel that repeated tapping is not necessary.
4. The baby should be handled as little as possible. Do not pick the infant up for feeding; if the baby is so weak that he cannot be fed while lying in the crib, parenteral feeding may be necessary. Gavage feeding may be necessary.

SUBDURAL HEMATOMA

The history is of utmost importance. The condition should be suspected in cases in which there were multiple births (prematurity), difficult deliveries, postnatal trauma, convulsions, vomiting (usually projectile), infection, failure to gain weight, hyperirritability, stupor, and evidence of retinal hemorrhage on funduscopic examination. The condition is not always a pediatric emergency but may become so when there is evidence of increased intracranial pressure manifested by projectile vomiting and convulsions.

The diagnosis is confirmed by subdural puncture and by this procedure alone; if the tap is positive, the removal of fluid is also the first step in treatment. The technique for subdural tap is described on page 210. Certain points may be emphasized with reference to other associated procedures.

COMA—Cont'd
SUBDURAL HEMATOMA—Cont'd

1. A spinal puncture should also be performed to rule out the possibility of a coexistent subarachnoid hemorrhage.
2. Daily subdural taps are usually performed with the removal of at least 10-12 c.c. of fluid each time until a negative tap is obtained. It is usually of practical importance to save the daily specimens for comparison with each other.
3. Neurosurgical intervention should be planned for the removal of the subdural membrane that is usually present.

EXTRADURAL HEMATOMA

The symptom complex produced by extradural hematoma in infancy and childhood varies considerably from the classical syndrome seen in adults. In children this is explained by the open sutures and fontanels, the greater elasticity of the cranial bones, and the increased frequency of venous bleeding rather than hemorrhage from the middle meningeal artery as the source of blood. Ingraham et al.[9] has reported 20 cases found among 1000 head injuries in children under 12 years of age, giving an incidence of 2%. A thorough knowledge of the special symptomatology of this lesion in pediatric practice is essential for only through prompt institution of neurosurgical therapy can the mortality rate be lowered.

Symptoms

The first symptoms are those produced by the effect of the trauma on the scalp and are usually pain and swelling.

The most important feature is the absence of initial unconsciousness immediately following the trauma in the great majority of patients. Instead there is a latent period between the trauma and the onset of stupor or neurological signs. With deepening of the stupor, hemiparesis and/or coma is likely to follow.

COMA—Cont'd
EXTRADURAL HEMATOMA—Cont'd
Symptoms—Cont'd

The blood lost from the general circulation in the formation of an extradural hematoma produces systemic effects in children not seen in adults. The loss of 100-150 c.c. of blood will produce profound shock in an infant, and amounts up to 400 c.c. have been obtained at operation.

Physical Signs

Ingraham[9] tabulates the following physical signs in order of their frequency:

1. Scalp swelling
2. Hemiparesis
3. Stupor
4. Positive Babinski reflex contralateral to hemiparesis and ipsilateral to lesions
5. Dilated pupil contralateral to hemiparesis and ipsilateral to lesion
6. Coma
7. Decerebrate posture
8. Convulsions
9. Strabismus
10. Papilledema

Laboratory Data

Blood counts will frequently demonstrate anemia due to blood loss; this is more marked in infants.

Lumbar puncture is not productive of constant findings but is of value in the differential diagnosis. The pressure, red blood cell count, and white blood cell count may be normal or elevated. The latter when elevated suggests the latent period has been sufficiently long to permit meningeal irritation.

X-ray of the skull will demonstrate cranial bone fracture and/or diastasis of the sutures in most instances.

COMA—Cont'd
EXTRADURAL HEMATOMA—Cont'd

Diagnosis

The occurrence of a latent period between the episode of head trauma and the development of symptoms and signs is the most important diagnostic feature in the clinical evaluation.

Further suspicion is justified if stupor and signs progress and there is a localized swelling of the scalp.

Definite diagnosis can only be established by trephination of the skull, and the above sequence of events warrants this procedure.

Treatment

Preoperative.

1. Immediate CBC, hematocrit, and typing and cross-matching for transfusion should be done. If condition will permit, a lumbar puncture should be performed.
2. Shock, if present, must be treated immediately and blood volume and quality restored.
3. All efforts should be directed to facilitate the earliest surgical intervention feasible.
4. On going to the operating room, the patient should have a cannula inserted via cut down in the saphenous vein and adequate fresh whole blood should be on hand.

Operative.

1. Trephination followed by bone flap operation and evacuation of hematoma.

Postoperative care.

1. General supportive therapy.
2. If initial spinal tap is bloody, daily taps are done until the RBC numbers less than 500 per cubic millimeter.
3. Lumbar puncture is performed for hyperthermia, and if the pressure is increased, it is reduced by ½ each time the lumbar puncture is performed.
4. Prophylactic antibiotic and chemotherapy.

References

1. Harris, R. C., et al.: The Treatment of Tetanus; Report of Two Cases With Critical Comment on New Therapeutic Resources, Pediatrics **2:** 175, 1948.
2. Queries and Minor Notes: J. A. M. A. **139:** 68, 1949.
3. Dodd, K.: Hypocalcemic States, Pediatrics **2:** 737, 1948.
4. Drake, M. E., et al.: Aureomycin in the Treatment of Influenzal Meningitis, J.A.M.A. **142:** 463, 1950.
4a. Bean, E. O., and Ross, S.: H. Influenzal Meningitis Treated With Aureomycin and Sulfadiazine, Clin. Proc. Child. Hosp. Wash. (D. C.) **6:** 1, 1949.
5. Kagan, B. M.: Influenzal Meningitis, Recovery of a Case of 4 Weeks' Duration With the Use of a New Drug, Polymyxin B (Aerosporin), Pediatrics **4:** 319, 1949.
6. Lincoln, E. M., and Kairmes, T. W: Streptomycin—Promizole Therapy of Miliary and Meningeal Tuberculosis in Children, Am. Rev. Tuberc. **61:** 159, 1950.
7. Almklov, J. R., and Hansen, A. E.: Aureomycin in Staphylococcic Meningitis Complicating Subarachnoid Hemorrhage in Sickle Cell Anemia, Pediatrics **3:** 764, 1949.
8. Hartmann, A., and Erganian, J.: Treatment of Diabetic Acidosis, J. Pediat. **31:** 274, 1947.
9. Ingraham, F., et al.: Extradural Hematoma in Infancy and Childhood, J.A.M.A. **140:** 1010, 1949.
10. Alexander, H. E.: The Treatment of Purulent Meningitides. In Advances in Pediatrics, vol. II, New York, 1947, Interscience Publishers, Inc.
11. Alexander, H. E.: Personal communication.
12. Colwell, A. R.: Diabetes Mellitus in General Practice, 1947, Chicago, The Year Book Publishers, Inc., pp. 240-250.

CHAPTER V

RESPIRATORY EMERGENCIES

Marked dyspnea is always a cause for anxiety, for the patient as well as for the physician, and requires early diagnosis and prompt therapy.

Since effective therapy depends frequently on anatomic localization, careful physical examination of the patient is necessary. The classical signs of laryngeal obstruction are retraction above the suprasternal notch and clavicles and below the xiphoid process. There is also frequently an inspiratory stridor with retraction of the intercostal spaces. When these signs are evident, several conditions should be considered:

- Croup
  - A. Specific (diphtheria)
  - B. Laryngotracheobronchitis
- Asthma
- Pneumonia
- Angioneurotic edema
- Acute bronchiolitis (pneumonitis in infancy)
- Foreign bodies and tumors

Other conditions necessitating emergency therapy because of respiratory difficulty are:

- Tracheo-esophageal fistula
- Respiratory paralysis due to central nervous system involvement, including poliomyelitis
- Asphyxia neonatorum and atelectasis
  - A. Massive atelectasis
- Pulmonary edema
- Pneumothorax*

*For a discussion of Mediastinal Emphysema, see addendum, page 235.

CROUP

A. SPECIFIC (Diphtheria)

Diphtheria should be suspected in all cases of croup and laryngotracheobronchitis. Smear and culture of nose and throat may rule out or confirm the diagnosis. (A rapid method for culturing the diphtheritic organism is available. It should be used as frequently as possible. A sterile cotton swab is dipped into normal horse serum and then flamed dry. If such a swab is used for diagnostic purposes, it should be incubated at body temperature for 4 hours. At this time if diphtheria is present the organism may be seen on smears taken from this culture). Even though culture fails to reveal a diphtheritic organism, adequate doses of diphtheria antitoxin must be given if there is a definite clinical impression of diphtheria. Such clinical impression may be based upon the following criteria, depending on the location of the diphtheritic membrane.

1. *Nasal.*
   (a) Like a "head cold."
   (b) Serosanguineous nasal discharge.
   (c) Nasal membrane.
   (d) Varying amounts of nasal hemorrhage, with associated irritation and inflammation of the upper lip.
2. *Pharyngeal.*
   There is fever, pain in the throat, exhaustion, and tachycardia increased out of proportion to a relatively low fever. Diphtheria membrane may involve tonsil pillars and soft palate, including uvula. The amount of blood in the membrane varies its color; it is markedly adherent to mucous membrane—bleeds when separated.
3. *Laryngeal.*
   Thinner membrane. Obstruction to breathing which may be (a) mechanical, (b) secondary to edema. Temperature may rise as high as 105°; cough is dry, tight; child shows anxiety and fear. Respiratory amplitude is increased and respirations forced.

CROUP—Cont'd
A. SPECIFIC (Diphtheria)—Cont'd

Treatment

1. Administration of diphtheria antitoxin.
   (a) The procedure for skin and ophthalmic testing as well as the procedure for the administration of diphtheria antitoxin should be that recommended in the section on Tetanus Antitoxin Administration (page 51).
   (b) If the patient proves to be sensitive to horse serum and if antitoxin is definitely indicated, an attempt should be made to desensitize* the patient to horse serum as outlined also in the section on Tetanus (page 52).

   IF THE CHILD IS SENSITIVE TO SERUM, THE ANTITOXIN MUST NEVER BE GIVEN INTRAVENOUSLY!

   (c) In mild or moderately severe cases, 25,000 to 50,000 units of antitoxin are given.
   (d) In severely ill patients, 50,000 to 100,000 units of antitoxin are given according to the severity of the infection. The intramuscular route is always the preferable route.
   (e) The total dose of antitoxin should be given in the first dose. If a second dose seems indicated later, it should be given soon after the first dose (within a few days—before serum sensitivity develops).
2. Penicillin in large doses should always be given, in addition, for bacteriostasis of the streptococcus which lives saprophytically with the diphtheria. The penicillin also, however, inhibits multiplication of diphtheria to a certain extent.
3. The patient with diphtheria must be kept at absolute bed rest for a period of not less than one month. Diph-

*True or complete desensitization is not actually possible. Nevertheless, practically speaking, the method outlined makes it possible to administer the antitoxin fairly safely.

CROUP—Cont'd
A. SPECIFIC (Diphtheria)—Cont'd
Treatment—Cont'd
3. Bed rest—Cont'd

theria myocarditis usually manifests itself in the third or fourth week of the illness, although death from early circulatory failure may occur as early as the eighth day. In this complication, the patient usually becomes restless and distressed. There may be vomiting and abdominal pain. Irregularities of rate and rhythm are observed. The pulse rate may fall if there is heart block or may rise suddenly with interference of vagus control. The heart sounds may become distant, poor in quality, and irregular.

4. According to Wilkens,[1] acute adrenal insufficiency may develop during acute diphtheria infections, especially with myocarditis. For this reason the judicious use of aqueous adrenal cortical extract is indicated as outlined on page 67.

B. LARYNGOTRACHEOBRONCHITIS

Laryngotracheobronchitis (croup), an infection of the laryngotracheobronchial tree, may be due to any one or any combination of the various bacteria or viruses. There is marked inflammation and varying amounts of edema of the mucosal tissue. This is frequently followed by relative laryngeal obstruction. The term "croup" is limited to those conditions where there is an associated relative stenosis. Most commonly, this is due to a supraglottic and, fortunately, less frequently to an infraglottic edema. Not uncommonly there is marked swelling of the surrounding lymphoid tissues, especially in the postlaryngeal area. This may be demonstrated in a lateral x-ray view of the neck where anterior displacement of the trachea can be observed.

The onset usually follows close upon a simple upper respiratory infection and often occurs very suddenly at night. There is respiratory difficulty, a brassy, barklike cough, and a

CROUP—Cont'd
B. LARYNGOTRACHEOBRONCHITIS—Cont'd

hoarse or absent voice. Fever may or may not be a prominent factor.

Treatment

This is a true medical emergency and requires immediate and definitive treatment.

1. If the patient is first seen at home, immediate transfer to the hospital must be accomplished, if possible. (If patient cannot be sent to the hospital, a steam room may be produced simply and efficiently in a closed bathroom by running hot water from shower or tap.) Tracheotomy, if needed, should be delayed whenever possible until this procedure can be done under controlled hospital conditions. En route to the hospital alternate exposure of the face to cold and warm atmosphere of air may temporarily partially reduce the edema and hence the relative asphyxia. If necessary, a Mosher Life-Saving Airway may be inserted. This may be accomplished by placing the child on his back with the head hanging a little lower than the rest of the body. The forefinger of one hand is used as a retractor and the tongue is pulled downward and forward. The airway is then slipped along the base of the tongue, using the retractor forefinger as a guide, and into the larynx. It must be realized that with the passing of the airway tube, the patient has been generally committed to a tracheotomy immediately upon hospital admission. Therefore, do not use the Mosher Life-Saving Airway unless absolutely necessary.
2. On admission to the hospital, the child should be placed in a steam cubicle or croup tent with continuous steam or in an oxygen tent with an attached humidifier. This is best accomplished by bubbling the oxygen through water before it enters the tent. Recent studies indicate

CROUP—Cont'd
B. LARYNGOTRACHEOBRONCHITIS—Cont'd
Treatment—Cont'd
2. Steam cubicle or croup tent—Cont'd

that moist oxygen* or cool moist air may produce a better effect more quickly than hot steam.

3. Nose and throat cultures with sensitivity of predominant organisms to the various antibiotics are then taken.
4. Start oral sulfadiazine and intramuscular penicillin at once. Streptomycin, Chloromycetin, or aureomycin may be later substituted or added when indicated, if the organism and its sensitivity to them is established.
5. Oxygen, penicillin aerosol, and streptomycin aerosol should be used as outlined:
   (a) Dissolve 50,000 units of potassium penicillin G in 0.5 c.c. of normal saline and mix with 25 mg. of streptomycin previously dissolved in 0.5 c.c. of normal saline.
   (b) Use ordinary aerosol nebulizer through which oxygen is allowed to flow at 6-8 liters per minute. Allow 3-4 minutes for complete treatment.
   (c) Use small hood for infants. Use small hood or Barach mask for older children.
   (d) Repeat treatment every 3 or 4 hours.
   Oxygen may be administered continuously during intervals between aerosol treatment.
6. Laryngoscopy on admission is no longer generally considered to be a routine procedure. It may be added that superimposed trauma accompanied by the secondary edema of this procedure may commit the patient to a tracheotomy.†
7. The patient should be allowed to have maximum rest and quiet. Constant handling is contraindicated. The patient, however, should be under constant observation for progressive asphyxia. The pulse rate, amplitude, and quality are especially important.

---

*Refer to use of oxygen tent and Croupette in the section on Pediatric Procedures, page 225.

†If a competent laryngoscopist is available, direct laryngoscopy may be useful for diagnostic as well as therapeutic purposes.

CROUP—Cont'd
B. LARYNGOTRACHEOBRONCHITIS—Cont'd
Treatment—Cont'd

8. With increasing asphyxia, increasing respiratory difficulty, and an irregular pulse, tracheotomy is the procedure of choice. Intubation is at present being discarded because of pathologic vocal cord changes associated with its prolonged use and because of the difficult nursing problems it presents.
9. Whiskey (1 dram to 1 ounce of sugar water) is the sedative of choice.
10. Parenteral hydration must be assured when oral intake of fluids is poor. Consideration must also be given to the extra loss of water from the body surface if the child is in a steam cubicle.

Posttracheotomy Care

1. Chevalier Jackson emphasizes "opiates and atropine should never be given this patient."
2. The tracheotomy tube should be aspirated frequently with a long, soft rubber catheter. The cannula is cleansed by pulling gauze, moistened with saline, through it with a piece of wire. It is dried by repeating the procedure with dry gauze.
3. Acidosis and dehydration must be watched for and treated.
4. Antibiotics should be given in full therapeutic dosage to prevent secondary infection of the respiratory tract.
5. A nurse must be in constant attendance.
6. Signs of cardiac failure must be anticipated. Weekly electrocardiograms should be taken to detect early T wave changes indicative of myocardial involvement.

ASTHMA

Dyspnea is most commonly caused by asthma. The symptoms are cough, wheezing, dyspnea, and a tightness in the

ASTHMA—Cont'd

chest. Auscultation generally reveals sibilant and sonorous râles most noticeable during expiration. There is usually a prolongation of the expiratory phase of respiration, and the pause usually heard between inspiration and expiration disappears.

Treatment

1. Adrenalin chloride in aqueous solution, 1:1000, 0.1 c.c. under 2 years of age; 0.2 c.c. over 2 years of age. Several small doses at intervals of 20 to 30 minutes are more effective and better tolerated than a single large dose.
2. Some asthmatics get greater relief by using Adrenalin in a 1:100 solution by means of a nebulizer. The plastic nebulizer is connected to a rubber bulb, which is squeezed as the patient inspires. One or two squeezes during each 3 to 5 inspirations will generally suffice.
3. The inhalation of steam or cold vapor may be of value in some persons with asthma. Many allergists now advocate unmedicated steam with sedation instead of large doses of adrenalin-type drugs.
4. Ephedrine sulfate may be given to older children in capsule form in oral doses of 3/16 gr. (0.015 Gm.) to 3/8 gr. (0.03 Gm.). A more satisfactory response is usually obtained when a barbiturate is given with the ephedrine.
5. Propadrine hydrochloride is sometimes tolerated better than ephedrine. This may be used in capsules of 3/16 gr. to 3/4 gr. orally, every 3 or 4 hours.
6. Aminophylline is often helpful in a prolonged attack. It may be given orally, intravenously, rectally, or by nebulizer. The following doses with individual method of administration are listed:
   (a) Orally—5-7½ gr. (0.30 to 0.5 Gm.) every 4 hours.
   (b) Intravenously—0.006 Gm. per kilogram in 10-20 c.c. of 10-25% dextrose in water. GIVE SLOWLY.

ASTHMA—Cont'd
Treatment—Cont'd
6. Aminophylline—Cont'd

(c) Rectally—0.125 Gm. every 4-6 hours in infants; 0.250 Gm. every 4 to 6 hours in older children.
(d) Nebulization—10-20 c.c. of 0.25 Gm. in an acute attack.

Many physicians feel that aminophylline is not very effective by the oral route. It is also felt that, because of the high alkalinity of the medication, the intramuscualr method should be discouraged because of its very irritating reaction. When given intravenously, it must be given very slowly and well diluted. Rectally, it may be given as a retention enema in 20 c.c. of tap water.

7. 100 to 300 c.c. of 25% glucose intravenously or 500 to 1000 c.c. of 10% glucose is sometimes an excellent supportive measure.
8. In a few cases where there is real status asthmaticus, ether in oil is sometimes necessary and of value. One-half to one ounce of ether mixed with an equal amount of warm olive oil is given by rectum. A smaller amount may be repeated every few hours for 24 hours.
9. Oxygen, with or without helium, is generally useful, but caution should be used in ordering a tent because these patients are generally too apprehensive.
   Positive pressure may diminish the inspiratory negative pressure, thus reducing the tendency to draw excessive mucus from the bronchial glands. It must be emphasized that the administration of positive pressure to children should be entrusted only to those trained in this type of therapy.
10. Antibiotics, including the sulfonamide group, penicillin, aureomycin, Chloromycetin, etc., should be used in full therapeutic dosage to prevent secondary infections or to treat concurrent infections.
11. Potassium iodide solution may be offered to liquify secretions which have become quite tenacious. Start with

ASTHMA—Cont'd
Treatment—Cont'd

1 drop t.i.d. and increase gradually to tolerance of the patient.

12. Various antihistamine agents have also been used. It may be stated that they have little, if any, effect in acute asthma when given orally. Recently,[1a] however, the use of aerosol antihistamine therapy has been attended with reasonable success in some cases. It certainly should be tried in the resistant cases.
13. These patients need a great deal of reassurance, attention, and encouragement. Psychologic consultation should be employed to help with the deeper psychosomatic aspects of the etiology of the asthmatic attacks.

PNEUMONIA

Since the advent of the sulfonamides and antibiotics, severe pneumonias in an emergency state are seldom encountered. However, occasionally a debilitated infant with a fulminating pneumonia may show severe cyanosis, dyspnea, circulatory collapse, acidosis, dehydration, and diarrhea. These require emergency treatment.

Treatment

1. Oxygen may be administered in a small tent in which the oxygen is humidified and cooled by passing through ice water. A Croupette is quite useful.*
2. Sulfadiazine, 1-1½ gr. per pound in 24 hours parenterally (as described in section on Meningitis, page 61).
3. Potassium penicillin G in aqueous solution (50,000 units every 3 hours intramuscularly) should also be administered. It may, however, also be given in single daily intramuscular injections of 300,000 units as procaine penicillin G in aqueous suspension.

---

*See section on Oxygen Therapy, page 225.

PNEUMONIA—Cont'd
Treatment—Cont'd

4. In primary atypical pneumonia aureomycin or Chloromycetin are the drugs of choice. Although optimum dosage schedules remain to be established, 20 to 50 mg. per kilogram per day generally prove adequate. This amount is usually given orally in divided doses but may be given rectally following a small cleansing enema in cases demonstrating gastrointestinal toxicity to the antibiotics. If extreme nausea or vomiting occurs, aureomycin may be given intravenously (see page 64).
5. Transfusion of plasma or whole blood is indicated for circulatory collapse.
6. If diarrhea develops during the course of a pneumonia, stop oral feedings and treat as outlined in section on Diarrhea (page 27).

FOREIGN BODIES AND TUMORS

Foreign bodies and tumors can produce respiratory obstruction. The diagnosis of foreign bodies requires a careful history, fluoroscopy, and x-ray of chest (posterior-anterior and lateral views of neck to show trachea), and laryngoscopic or bronchoscopic examination.

Treatment

1. Removal of foreign body by a competent bronchoscopist.
2. Oxygen may be used following removal because of laryngeal edema due to bronchoscopic procedure.
3. Antibiotics, to control secondary infection, should be started immediately.

Tumors will require surgery through the bronchoscope or open thoracic surgery.

ANGIONEUROTIC EDEMA

(See Section on Serum Sickness, page 177)

TRACHEO-ESOPHAGEAL FISTULA

Another condition that may be considered a respiratory emergency in the newborn period is tracheo-esophageal fistula. Although the therapy of this condition is essentially and ultimately surgical, its diagnosis depends on careful history.

Symptoms of coughing, sputtering, cyanosis, and dyspnea usually occur *at the first oral feeding.* Should these occur, careful examination, both physical and roentgenologic, should be made to determine the presence of this anomaly before more feedings are given. *Any difficulty with the first oral feeding in the newborn should be reported by the nurse to the attending physician immediately.*

Management

1. Stop all oral feedings.
2. Institute oropharyngeal suction.
3. Order postural drainage.
4. Parenteral fluid therapy is essential.
5. Therapeutic doses of penicillin are helpful and should be requested.
6. Surgical consultation should be requestetd as soon as radiologic diagnosis is established. The first step in diagnosis should be the introduction of a small rubber catheter into the esophagus under direct fluoroscopic visualization. If obstruction is encountered, ½ to 1 c.c. of Lipiodol should be introduced into the esophageal pouch through a small catheter. *BARIUM SHOULD NEVER BE USED.*

One postoperative complication may be anticipated; namely, laryngeal stridor with temporary cardiac and respiratory arrest. In some instances,[2] laryngeal stridor coming on during or shortly after feeding has been noted in the early postoperative period. This is thought to be due to excessive vagal activity.

(a) The administration of atropine sulfate is indicated. Start with 1 drop of a 1:2000 atropine sulfate solution (0.0003 Gm.) 10 minutes a.c. Increase this amount gradually to tolerance.

ACUTE BRONCHIOLITIS (PNEUMONITIS) OF INFANCY

The severe phase of acute bronchiolitis is fairly frequently encountered in pediatric practice, especially in infants under 6 months of age. It is ushered in with a frequent, distressing cough associated with an audible wheeze. The patient generally appears apathetic and is obviously seriously ill. The temperature ranges from 102° to 103°. There is always a rapid pulse and frequently a very rapid respiratory rate (as high as 60 to 80 per minute) associated with marked dyspnea. Many râles may be heard throughout the lung fields.

Treatment

Therapy should be promptly directed toward control of infection, respiratory distress with associated oxygen lack, and circulatory collapse.

1. Sulfadiazine should be given orally in doses of 1 to 1½ gr. per pound per day in divided doses.
2. Penicillin should be administered in doses of 50,000 units every 3 hours intramuscularly.
3. Dihydrostreptomycin or streptomycin should be administered in doses of 20 mg. per pound per day in divided doses given every 12 hours.
4. Penicillin and streptomycin should also be given in the form of aerosol treatment as outlined in the section on Laryngotracheobronchitis (page 84).
5. Aureomycin should be administered in doses of 20 to 40 mg. per kilogram per day in divided doses, given every 6 hours.
6. High concentrations of moist oxygen should be administered.
7. Bronchiolar spasm and edema of lungs and central nervous system may be affectively managed with the intravenous administration of aminophylline (0.006 Gm. per kilogram) in 50% dextrose (2 c.c. per kilogram). This

ACUTE BRONCHIOLITIS (PNEUMONITIS) OF INFANCY—Cont'd
Treatment—Cont'd

7. Bronchiolar spasm and edema of lungs and C.N.S.—Cont'd

amount should be given slowly intravenously every 6 or 8 hours, as indicated, to control dyspnea.

8. Careful symptomatic treatment is also essential:
   (a) Adequate nursing care is essential.
   (b) Only clear fluids should be given by mouth until patient has recovered from marked dyspnea and tachypnea.
   (c) Parenteral fluids should be given to maintain fluid and electrolyte balance. Special emphasis should be placed on avoiding excess sodium ion administration. Thus, 5% or 10% dextrose in distilled water, plasma, and whole blood should be the mainstays of treatment in the acute period.
   (d) Abdominal distention must be relieved by one or a combination of the following methods:
      (1) Warmth to abdomen, rectal tube, or small enema.
      (2) Prostigmine Methylsulfate, 0.25 to 1.0 c.c. of a 1:4000 solution subcutaneously.
      (3) Pitressin, 0.5 to 1.5 units intramuscularly.
   (e) If respiratory depression occurs, caffeine sodium benzoate, ½ to 2 gr., may be used intravenously. It should be avoided, however, in the stage of respiratory hyperactivity.
   (f) If cardiac failure becomes imminent, prompt digitalization may be of distinct value.
   (g) If the diagnosis of pertussis is suggested by either history or character of the cough, early use of hyperimmune pertussis serum is indicated—at least until pertussis is definitely eliminated as a possibility. In the very sick infant 20 c.c. of the lyophilized human pertussis serum (Philadelphia Serum Exchange) may be given intravenously.

RESPIRATORY PARALYSIS IN POLIOMYELITIS*

TABLE VII. SUMMARY OF SYMPTOMS AND TREATMENT IN VARIOUS TYPES OF BULBAR POLIOMYELITIS

(Compiled from Bulbar Form of Poliomyelitis, Minn. Polio. Res. Comm., J. A. M. A., 1947,[3] and from Baker: Bulbar Poliomyelitis, Am. J. Med., 1949.[4])

SYMPTOMS	TREATMENT
I. Bulbar-Cranial Nerve Nuclei Group	
1. Difficulty in swallowing 2. Regurgitation of food and fluids through nose (particularly in children)	Parenteral feeding, nasal feeding
3. Pooling of secretions in throat (salivation?) 4. Nasal speech, hoarseness, inability to talk	Impending obstruction of airway Postural drainage, suction, elective tracheotomy
5. Stridor, dyspnea, cyanosis (obstructed airway)	Emergency intubation and/or tracheotomy
6. Anxiety and restlessness (hypoxia)	Oxygen therapy, tent, mask, ets., humidified
7. Other cranial nerve involvements, opthalmoplegias, facial palsies	No treatment necessary
II. Bulbar-Respiratory Center Group	
1. Adequate function of respiratory muscles 2. Adequate airway	
3. Variations in rate and depth of respirations (impending failure; observe carefully) 4. Prolonged intervals between respirations 5. Anxiety, restlessness, increasing pulse rate (hypoxia)	Oxygen therapy (elective tracheotomy)
6. Increasing periods of apnea 7. Confusion, delirium, pulmonary congestion (anoxia) 8. Cyanosis	Tracheotomy Respirator Intensive oxygen therapy with positive pressure, if possible; sedation with extreme caution
III. Bulbar-Circulatory Center Group	
1. Dusky red, flushed, florid appearance	Intensive oxygen therapy (tracheotomy, if indicated)
2. Rapid (150-200) pulse 3. Irregular, thready pulse 4. Elevated blood pressure; decreased pulse pressure 5. Anxiety; restlessness 6. Shocklike state (falling blood pressure, imperceptible pulse) 7. Cold, clammy, mottled cyanosis 8. Hyperthermia, delirium, coma	Supportive measures
IV. Bulbar-Encephalitic Group	
1. Hyperexcitability 2. Restlessness and anxiety 3. Muscular tremors and twitchings 4. Confusion and irritability 5. Lethargy, somnolence, and coma 6. Convulsions (chiefly in children)	Intensive oxygen therapy: Mask Tent Intranasal oxygen Tracheotomy, if indicated
V. Bulbar-Cervical Cord Group	
1. Cranial nerve palsies (see group I) 2. Symptoms of cardiorespiratory center involvement (see groups II and III) 3. Diaphragm and intercostal involvement	Early tracheotomy Intensive oxygen therapy Respirator

In addition, general prophylactic (antibiotic) and supportive therapy should be initiated at once.

*Electrophrenic respiration is referred to in the addendum, page 234.

ASPHYXIA NEONATORUM AND ATELECTASIS

A. Use postural drainage and suction if mucus is present.

B. Use oxygen.

C. Stimulation to breathing can sometimes be accomplished by rectal stimulation. In severe cases follow methods of resuscitation outlined on page 97.

D. Cardiorespiratory stimulant if heart rate is slow and/or markedly irregular: 0.2-0.4 c.c. of alpha-lobeline intravenously (use the longitudinal sinus or external jugular vein) or directly into the heart.

E. Prevention of asphyxia.

Recently[5] a method of preventing asphyxia in newborn infants delivered by caesarean section has been recommended. This method is suggested because of the observation that copious amounts of amniotic fluid may be found in the stomach of newborn infants delivered by section.

1. Gastric suction is done within a few minutes after birth. A No. 10 French catheter is passed slowly through the mouth with constant negative pressure from a resuscitator. After the stomach is reached, the abdomen is gently pressed.
2. Suction is applied during withdrawal of the catheter.
3. Oxygen is administered for 1- to 2-minute periods during the intervals between successive gastric suction.
4. Suction is repeated 2 or 3 times until no fluid is obtained.
5. The infant is placed in an oxygen-supplied incubator.
6. Mucus should be aspirated from the nasal pharynx as frequently as necessary.
7. Repeat gastric suction every 3 hours for 12 hours.

MASSIVE ATELECTASIS

Symptoms and Signs

1. Marked dyspnea.
2. Tachycardia.

ASPHYXIA NEONATORUM AND ATELECTASIS—Cont'd
MASSIVE ATELECTASIS—Cont'd
Symptoms and Signs—Cont'd

3. Cyanosis.
4. General prostration.
5. Pain in chest.
6. Chest appears flat on affected side and relatively immobile.
7. Heart and lungs displaced toward affected side.
8. Elevation of diaphragm on affected side.

Treatment

1. If unilateral, place child on unaffected side.
2. Slap chest.
3. Initiate crying or coughing.
4. Bronchoscopic aspirations are occasionally necessary.

PULMONARY EDEMA

This condition is not seen too frequently in infancy and childhood but its development must be anticipated in a variety of other conditions.

1. Severely toxic individuals with systemic infections.
2. Acute and chronic nephritis.
3. Heart failure in acute or chronic rheumatic heart disease.
4. Poisoning.
   (a) Barbiturates.
   (b) Carbon monoxide gas, chlorine, bromine, sulfur dioxide.
5. Inadvertent overhydration with parenteral fluids, especially in infancy.

Symptoms and Signs

Symptoms and signs may be variable but the following are quite constant:

1. Cyanosis (except in carbon monoxide poisoning).
2. Productive cough. Usually a blood-tinged, frothy sputum is seen (except in the small child).

PULMONARY EDEMA—Cont'd
Symptoms and Signs—Cont'd

3. Rapid but weak pulse.
4. Numerous, moist râles throughout lung fields.

Treatment

1. Eliminate cause, if known.
2. Specific antidote for known poisons.
3. Heart failure or nephritis, if present, should be promptly treated as outlined in other sections of this book (pages 17 and 37).
4. Oxygen in high concentrations.
5. Morphine may have some distinct value. A safe dose for various ages is presented in the section on Preanesthetic Medication (page 176).

PNEUMOTHORAX

Pneumothorax is a relatively rare condition during childhood. It does, however, occur occasionally in the newborn period and the symptoms may be alarming, depending upon the extent of the collapse of the lung and the position of the mediastinum. If the diagnosis is made or suspected, it should be confirmed by x-ray or fluoroscopic examination. The treatment will depend upon the cause, the severity of the symptoms, and the presence or absence of a communicating fistula.

1. Oxygen for dyspnea and cyanosis.
2. If infection is present, the use of antibiotic and/or sulfonamides is indicated, depending on the organism.
3. Where there is no fistula present and the symptoms are mild, the air will usually be absorbed in a week to ten days, and no further treatment is necessary.
4. If there are progressively increasing symptoms of pressure, the air should be aspirated as necessary.
5. If a communicating fistula is present, the aspiration of air should be omitted as long as possible to permit healing and closure of the opening.

PNEUMOTHORAX—Cont'd

6. On rare occasions it may be necessary to insert a blunt needle into the pleural space with an attachment to a water bottle, having the tube 1-2 cm. under water. This apparatus may be left attached for periods ranging from 2-4 hours to several days.

RESUSCITATION OF THE NEWBORN INFANT

Asphyxia neonatorum may be the result of many causes which can occur in utero, during delivery, or after birth. The anoxia may be of varying degrees of duration and severity. Failure to establish normal respiration at birth may continue pre-existing anoxia or initiate extrauterine anoxia.

The degree of asphyxia shown by the newborn infant at birth has been classified as follows:[6]

1. *Mild asphyxia.* There is absence of respiration in the first 30 seconds after birth of the head. Muscle tone is present. There is resistance to opening the mouth. Conjunctival and gag reflexes are elicited. The heart rate is rapid or normal.
2. *Moderate asphyxia.* There is poor or absent muscle tone and no resistance on opening the mouth. Aspiration or stimulation of the glottis causes no reflex irritation. The heart rate is rapid and may then become slow.
3. *Severe asphyxia.* There is no response to stimulation. Lividity or pallor may be present. There may be occasional or no cardiac impulse detectable.

In management of the asphyxiated infant, the effort to produce adequate respirations needs to be done quickly and safely. The following equipment should be available in the delivery room:

1. Some method of suction which may be a mechanical apparatus or a small catheter with mucus trap for suction by mouth.

RESUSCITATION OF NEWBORN INFANT—Cont'd

2. An infant laryngoscope, a No. 12 French, woven silk whistle tip, tracheal catheter, and the Flagg Resuscitation Apparatus* or other resuscitation devices with which the operator is familiar may be used.
3. Oxygen supply with suitable equipment for its administration.
4. A hypodermic set and stimulants such as caffeine sodium benzoate, epinephrine, and alpha-lobeline. Difference of opinion exists as to their effectiveness and possible dangers.

Failure of spontaneous onset of respirations or inadequate respiration will cause asphyxia. If breathing does not start within 30 seconds of birth, the infant is considered mildly asphyxiated. The condition of the asphyxiated infant does not remain static. There will be either improvement or progression to more severe degrees of asphyxia. Haste is imperative because complete anoxia of more than 2 or 3 minutes may cause irreparable damage to the brain. Treatment of the anoxia may require initiation of respirations, the production of more efficient breathing or the addition of more oxygen to the inspired air. Provision of warmth for the asphyxiated infant is important, and the baby should be placed in a heated crib. A minimum of handling is essential, and the baby should not be subjected to the trauma of manual artificial respiration. The cord is allowed to continue pulsating so as to deliver additional oxygen-carrying blood.

The following procedures are meanwhile being instituted:

1. Provision of clear airway to the lungs.
2. The airway may contain excess mucus, excess amniotic fluid, vernix, meconium, blood, and occasionally inflammatory exudate. It should be remembered that with the first breath taken by the normal newborn some tracheal and bronchial fluid, normal in the air pas-

*Hospital Model No. MR3, The Foregger Company, Inc., New York, N. Y.

RESUSCITATION OF NEWBORN INFANT—Cont'd

sage at birth, is drawn into the alveoli. With expansion of the lungs there will be sufficient space to take care of a normal amount of a mixture of mucus and amniotic fluid with facility largely by absorption through the capillaries of the alveolar walls. However, such substances as blood, vernix, inflammatory exudates, and meconium act as foreign bodies. At the birth of the infant and preferably before the first inspiration, the mouth, nose, and laryngopharynx can be cleared by postural drainage, gentle cleansing with gauze, and by suction. In mild asphyxia this toilet of the upper airway may act as a reflex to stimulate respiration. If there is no resistance to depressing the lower jaw, exposure of the laryngopharynx with the laryngoscope can be done. These recommendations presume some experience and familiarity with the infant laryngoscope, tracheal aspiration, and tracheal insufflation, using for the latter procedure the Flagg resuscitation apparatus. Practice in these procedures can be very satisfactorily carried out on stillborn infants. If on laryngoscopy active spasm of the glottis is seen, tracheal intubation will not be required as a respiratory effort can be anticipated. Clearing of the upper airway will provide adequate treatment. If, however, laryngoscopy shows the pharyngeal reflex to be absent and the vocal cords inactive, tracheal aspiration is indicated with the No. 12 catheter referred to above or other comparable infant suction tube introduced ½ to 1 inch into the trachea under direct visualization.

(The infant is showing the flaccidity of moderate or severe asphyxia.)

With the lower airway having been cleared and the infant still apneic, and the tracheal catheter still in place, the next step is, by tracheal insufflation to sup-

RESUSCITATION OF NEWBORN INFANT—Cont'd

ply oxygen to the lungs under intermittent slight pressure. Pure oxygen is delivered to the lungs at a pressure not greater than 12 inches of water by means of the Flagg apparatus. This has a safety blow-off mechanism which can be set so as not to exceed the water pressure desired. It is to be noted that pressure must never be permitted to build up over a period of more than 5 seconds. Adequate time should be allowed to permit expiration or deflation.

In brief summary, in moderate or severe asphyxiation one employs direct laryngoscopy, tracheal suction, and tracheal insufflation with the tube connected to pressure-controlled oxygen delivered to the lungs. The provision of oxygen by this mechanical resuscitative method should be continued until the infant is making reasonably good respiratory response of his own and has a good color. The infant is then placed in an incubator with oxygen and observed frequently and carefully. No feeding is to be offered for the first 12 to 18 hours. Several recent articles reported on the value of gastric suction at birth in infants delivered by cesarean section from diabetic mothers and likewise indicated its possible equal effectiveness in cesarean-born infants from nondiabetic mothers. It is considered that this procedure prevents significantly regurgitation of the stomach contents and its aspiration into the lungs. In view of the above favorable reports it would appear advisable to employ, in addition to the resuscitation measures listed above, gastric suction in the moderate and severely asphyxiated infant as a prophylaxis for subsequent regurgitation and aspiration into the lungs of stomach contents. This procedure is outlined in another section (page 94).

In the absence of trained personnel, reliance must be placed on postural drainage with gentle milking of the trachea and simple catheter suction of the nose, mouth, and laryngopharynx. Passing a catheter into the glottis by blind intuba-

RESUSCITATION OF NEWBORN INFANT—Cont'd

tion for tracheal aspiration recommended by some is less desirable and in reality may only be esophageal suction. Mouth-to-mouth insufflation is employed by some where mechanical facilities for resuscitation are not available. The Kreiselman resuscitator has an adjustable safety or "blow-off" feature whereby intermittent oxygen can be supplied by controlled pressure with the use of a face mask. It is important that the operator be familiar with the method of resuscitation employed. For the moderate and severely asphyxiated infant the same fundamental principles apply, no matter what method of resuscitation is used; namely, a minimum of handling, clearing the airway, provision of warmth, and supplying oxygen to the lungs under slight pressure.

SMOKE INHALATION

The effects of smoke inhalation may occasionally be as severe as actual burns. In addition, it may be as difficult to treat as are burns. The onset of symptoms may be delayed for several hours.

It is necessary to have knowledge of the symptoms of smoke inhalation. On the basis of experience gained by the staff of the Massachusetts General Hospital, the following 3 stages may generally be recognized:[7]

1. *Stage of excitement.*

   Hysteria, pain, and anoxia generally cause the marked hyperactivity.

   Treatment.

   (a) Small doses of intravenous Nembutal are most useful for the hysteria.

   (b) Small doses of intravenous morphine are most useful for the control of pain.

   (c) Anoxia should be treated by adequate oxygen administration through the proper airway.

SMOKE INHALATION—Cont'd

2. *Stage of edema of respiratory tract.*

   This stage generally develops about 24 hours after exposure.

   Symptoms and Signs.

   Cyanosis, dyspnea, restlessness, moist râles, edema, and inflammation of the larynx.

   Treatment.

   (a) Avoid saline and all parenteral fluids.
   (b) Laryngeal intubation or tracheotomy may be necessary.
   (c) Oxygen in high concentrations is valuable.

3. *Stage of bronchiolitis or pneumonitis.*

   Full doses of antibiotics are indicated because of the focal atelectasis, localized lobular collapse, and the bronchiolar constriction generally seen in this stage.

References

1. Jacobsen, A. W., et al.: Panel Discussion on the Adrenal Gland in Health and Disease, Pediatrics **3:** 546, 1949.
1a Rubitsky, H. J., et al.: Parenteral and Aerosol Administration of Antihistamine Agents in the Treatment of Severe Bronchial Asthma, New England J. Med. **241:** 853, 1949.
2. Mercer, R. D.: Laryngeal Stridor and Temporary Cardiorespiratory Arrest, Am. J. of Dis. Child. **70:** 336, 1941.
3. Bulbar Form of Poliomyelitis. II. Therapeutic Measures Based on Pathological and Physiological Findings, Minn. Polio. Res. Comm., J.A.M.A. **135:** 425, 1947.
4. Baker, A. B.: Bulbar Poliomyelitis, Am. J. Med. **6:** 614, 1949.
5. Gellis, S. A., et al.: Gastric Suction: A Proposed Additional Technique for the Prevention of Asphyxia in Infants Delivered by Caesarean Section, New England J. Med. **240:** 533, 1949.
6. Flagg, P. J.: The Art of Resuscitation, New York, 1944, Reinhold Publishing Company.
7. Orr, W., et al.: A Case of Smoke Inhalation, Clin. Proc. Child. Hosp. Wash. (D. C.) **5:** 342, 1949.

Other References on Resuscitation in the Newborn Not Referred to Specifically in the Text

Smith, C. A.: Effects of Birth Processes and Obstetrical Procedures Upon the Newborn Infant, in Advances in Pediatrics, New York, 1948, Interscience publishers, vol. 3.
Clifford, S. H.: Fetal Anoxia at Birth and Cyanosis of the Newborn, Amer. J. Dis. Child. **76:** 666, 1948.
Russ, J. D., and Strong, R. A.: Asphyxia of the Newborn Infant, Am. J. Obst. & Gynec. **51:** 643, 1946.

CHAPTER VI

DROWNING

Introduction

Although considerable progress was made in decreasing the number of fatal drownings in the period following World War I,[1] "there was little change in the annual rate of these fatalities in the ten-year period ending in 1947."[2] Drowning is the third largest cause of accidental death and claims approximately 6500 lives per year in the United States.[1-4] The success of any water-safety and first-aid program depends upon active and vigorous participation of our profession.

Treatment

Artificial Respiration

The most important single factor in the treatment of drowning is artificial respiration. Ample evidence has been adduced from many sources to demonstrate the vital importance of prompt institution of artificial respiration regardless of the method employed. Fig. 1[5] aptly demonstrates that the delay of 4-5 minutes after the cessation of spontaneous respiration appreciably lowers the chances of the victim's survival. Thus, this form of therapy should be started immediately upon removal of the victim from the water, whether he is on shore, in a lifeboat, on a raft, or in an airplane; the lapse of time between "landing" the drowner and reaching shore may prove fatal.

The operator or operators should first ascertain that there are no foreign bodies present in the oral cavity and that the tongue has not prolapsed posteriorly and then treatment is started, the delay being no more than 10 seconds. Artificial respiration must be continued until the absolute signs of death have appeared, in some instances 6 to 8 hours. The physician should be extremely cautious in pronouncing death and allowing treatment to stop, for amazing recoveries have

Treatment—Cont'd
Artificial Respiration—Cont'd

been reported. The ordinary signs of death such as the absence of audible heart sounds stethoscopically, peripheral pulse beat, respiratory excursion, and blood pressure are completely undependable[6, 7] in drowning. The absolute signs of death such as livor mortis, rigor mortis, and persistent hypothermia are the only reliable signs.

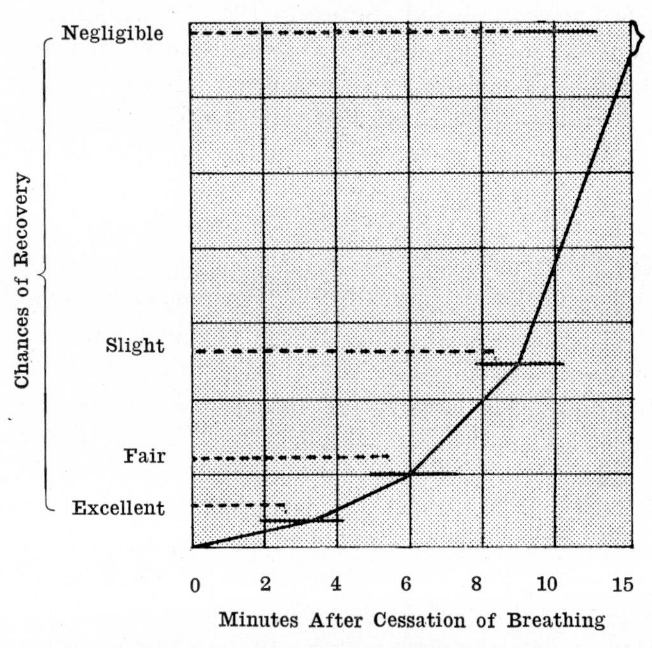

Fig. 1.—Graph of chances of survival after cessation of spontaneous breathing. It is assumed that a healthy adult stops breathing at 0. The chances of restoring resuscitations by appropriate measures are indicated by broken line. (Courtesy of Consolidated Edison Co., New York, N. Y.)

It is to be stressed that the adjuvant methods of therapy, to be discussed, should not be considered until artificial respiration has been started and should be carried out by an assistant in such a manner as to produce no hindrance to the operator.

Treatment—Cont'd

Warmth

The nearly drowned patient is uniformly in shock, and this is more severe if the suffocation has occurred in cold water. The cervical ganglion cells have a definite high and low thermal tolerance which when exceeded even minutely produces a complete paralysis which is reversible with the appropriate decrease or increase of temperature.[8] It is common experience that resuscitation is easier to accomplish when drowning has occured in warm water in contradistinction to the difficulties encountered when the victim has been in cold water.

The patient should be placed on a blanket when possible and covered, leaving exposed those parts necessary to accomplish treatment. Hot-water bottles or chemical heating pads (which generate heat on moistening) should be placed in the axillae and between the thighs.

Warm enemas should be given when possible.

Stimulants

Caffeine[9] is recommended as the best stimulant and should be administered parenterally,[10] preferably intravenously. The dose of caffeine sodium benzoate is 60-90 mg. per 10 kilograms of body weight and may be repeated in 30 minutes if necessary. Caffeine is indicated in all persons who are not conscious when seen by the physician. Amyl nitrite[11] is also of value in augmenting coronary circulation and is easily administered by crushing the perle and allowing the patient to "inhale" the drug in the course of artificial respiration. The use of epinephrine is not considered efficacious by most investigators.[6,9,11]

Oxygen

Inhalation of oxygen during artificial respiration is valuable in all cases. Care should be taken that the exhalation valve of the mask is open. If the mask is not equipped with such a valve, then it should not be held tightly on the face but just close to the mouth and nose.

Treatment—Cont'd
Oxygen—Cont'd

The use of carbon dioxide in combination with oxygen is considered valueless or even harmful.[12]

Respiration Devices

Any mechanical apparatus which attempts to insufflate the lungs with oxygen by positive pressure and then stimulate expiration by negative pressure is contraindicated in the treatment of the nearly drowned patient. Such machines may cause pulmonary collapse, atelectasis, or overdistention of the lungs.[9,13] It is impossible to regulate any one machine to conform with the vital capacities and respiratory cycles of all patients[14]; the latter is especially true of children.

Massage

Massage of the limbs, the stroke being toward the heart, may be of some value in stimulating circulation.

Bed Rest

The recently resuscitated patient should be kept at absolute bed rest and under constant observation for 24-48 hours. Where possible the individual should be hospitalized but only after spontaneous respirations have been established for at least 1-2 hours. The pulse, respirations, and blood pressure should be observed frequently for the first 24 hours because of the possibility of delayed shock.

Routine antibiotic administration is advisable as a prophylaxis against pneumonitis.

Frequent small sips of warm (not hot) liquids should be given followed by the gradual institution of a soft diet.

Methods of Artificial Respiration

The aims of artificial respiration are twofold—to foster ventilation and circulation—the former by producing an adequate exchange of gases in the pulmonary alveoli and the latter by stimulating cardiac output and venous return.

Methods of Artificial Respiration—Cont'd

There are two prominent methods in use today; i.e., the Schäfer Prone Pressure Method and The Eve Rocking Method. The Schäfer method has received wide acclaim and is the prominent method in the United States at this time. The Eve method has been received enthusiastically in England and has been preferentially adopted by the Royal Navy.[15] Both methods will be described.

Schäfer Prone Pressure Method

This procedure consists of the manual compression of the lower thoracic cage which decreases the intrathoractic volume and forces the diaphragm upward. It depends on the principle that on the release of this pressure, "the elasticity of the chest and abdomen cause these to resume their original dimensions and air passes in through the trachea."[16]

The standard technique is as follows:

1. The patient is laid on his abdomen with one arm extended and the other arm flexed at a right angle. The head is turned toward the extended arm so that the mouth and nose are free, and the head rests on the hand and forearm of the flexed arm. If the patient is on a declining plane, the body should be placed on the slope with the head lowermost.
2. The operator kneels straddling the patient's thighs facing forward and at such a distance from the patient's hip bones that he can place his hands on the patient's lower thorax with simple extension of his arms and without straining. The operator's palms are placed on the thorax so that his fifth finger lies along the lowest rib with the rest of the fingers in a natural position, their tips being just out of his sight along the lateral curvature of the chest. (Fig. 2.)
3. The operator then rocks forward, gradually bringing his weight to bear on the patient's chest, keeping his arms straight. At the end of this forward motion the opera-

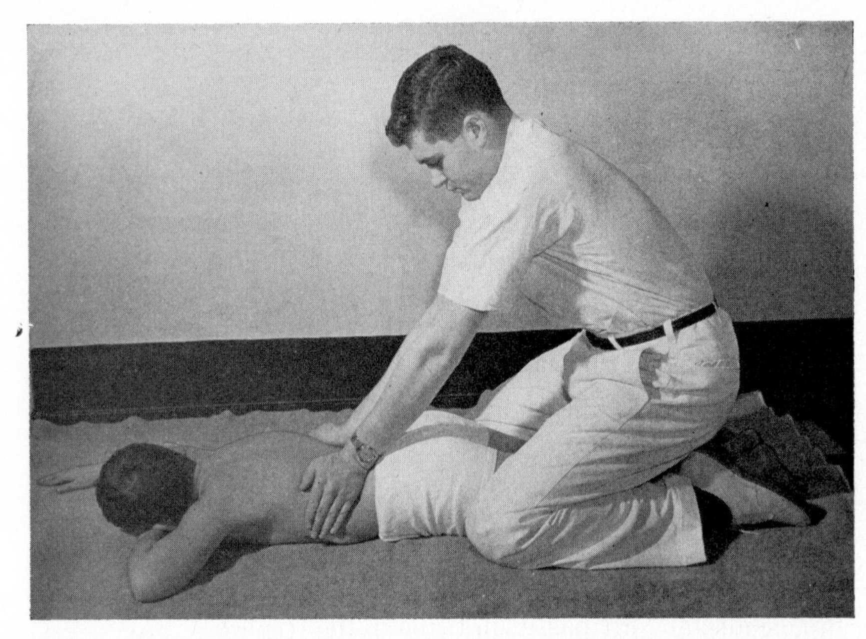

Fig. 2.—Operator ready to begin prone pressure artificial respiration. First maneuver.

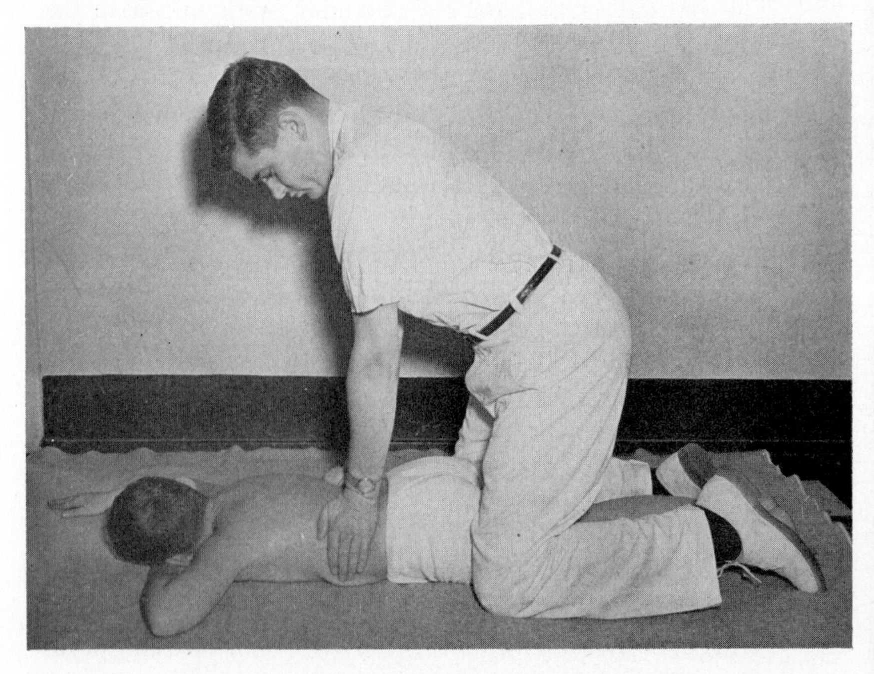

Fig. 3.—Artificial respiration. Second maneuver.

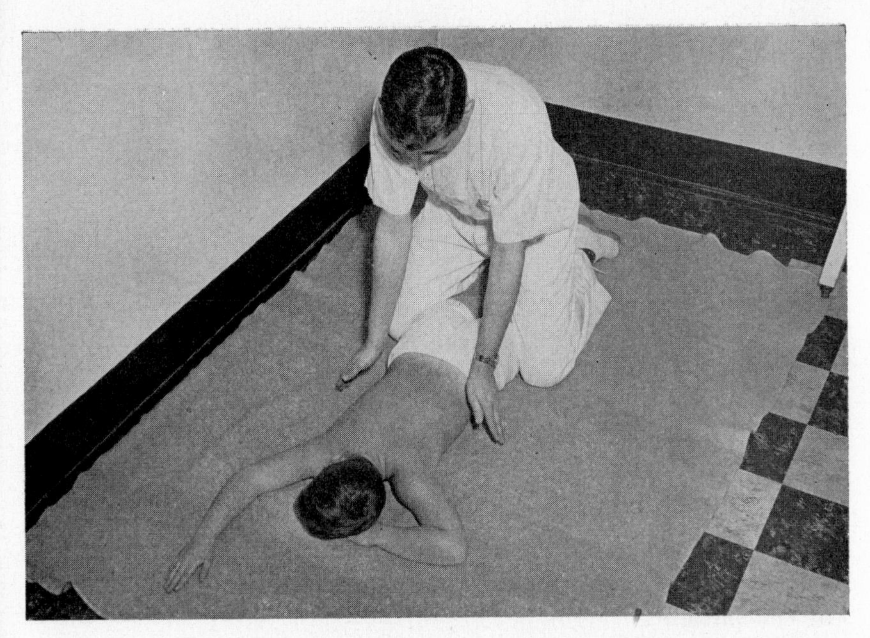

Fig. 4.—Artificial respiration. Third maneuver.

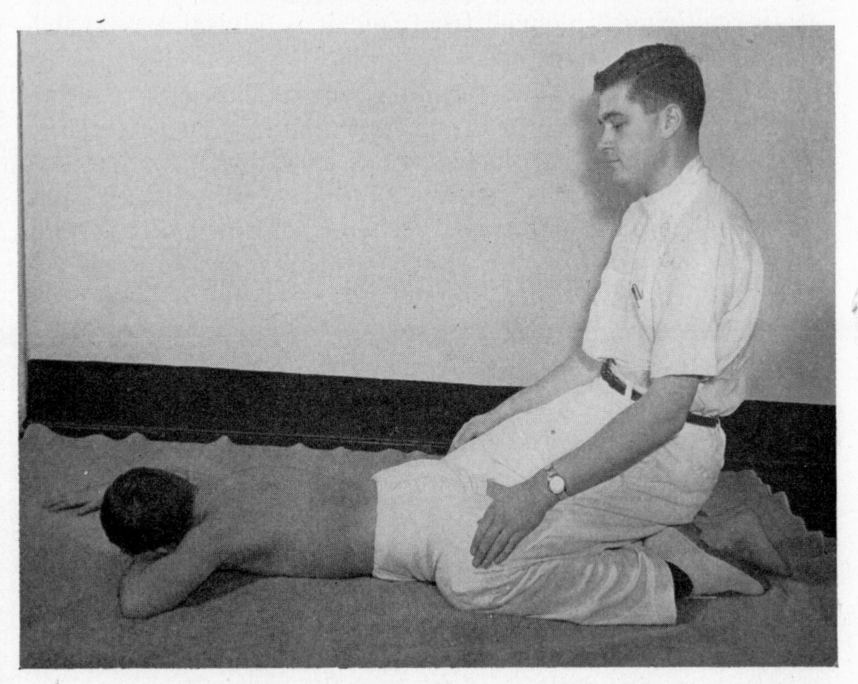

Fig. 5.—Artificial respiration. Fourth maneuver.

tor's shoulders are directly over the heels of his hands. (Fig. 3.) This phase occupies 2 seconds' time from placing of hands to the end of the forward swing.

4. The operator immediately releases his hands when at the zenith of the swing (Fig. 4) and returns to the resting position with his arms at his sides (Fig. 5). In 2 seconds the cycle is repeated.

   This should be done rhythmically and with a count, placing hands with 1, rocking with 2, releasing with 3, and resting with 4.

Naturally the amount of the operator's weight that is applied to the thorax should vary according to the size and age of the patient.

The operator's comfort must be considered and in those cases requiring prolonged treatment it is advisable to switch operators if substitutes are available. This is done in the following manner. The second operator kneels at the patient's side and gets into rhythm with the first operator (Fig. 6 . Then at the end of one cycle the substitute gives the next cycle while kneelin beside the patient, during which time the first operator withdraws. Then at the end of the next cycle the second operator straddles the knees and continues the treatment (Fig. 7).

This method can be used effectively by a single operator and should not be interrupted while transporting the victim. It is effective on the stern seat of a lifeboat, on a raft, or in an airplane. Members of a good team can move the patient and operator up the beach to escape the incoming tide without missing a stroke by dragging them on a blanket a few feet during the resting phase of each cycle.

Eve Rocking Method

Eve points out that in the nearly drowned patient there is a progressive failure of tone of the respiratory muscles

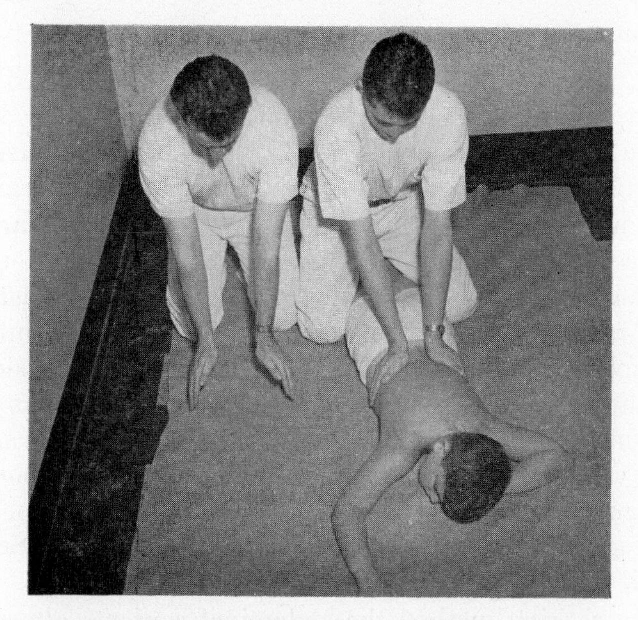

Fig. 6.—Artificial respiration. Fifth maneuver.

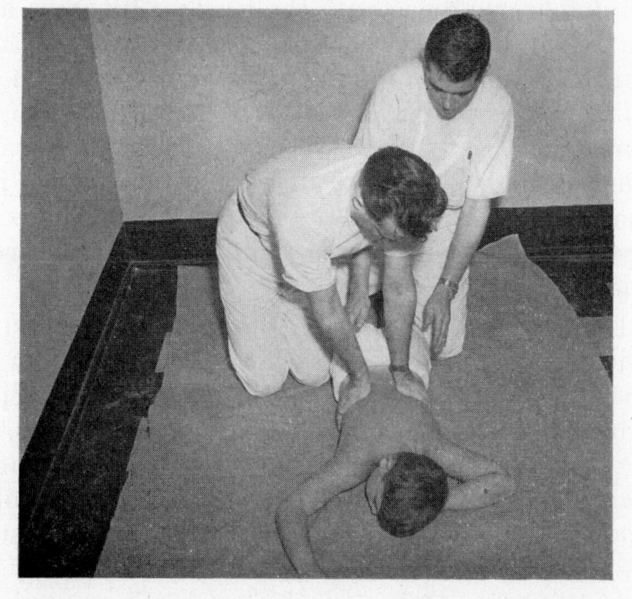

Fig. 7.—Artificial respiration. Sixth maneuver.

and diaphragm which is directly proportioned to the degree and the duration of anoxia.[17] This produces a constantly increasing hindrance to the elastic recoil of the thorax and abdomen (on release of manual compression) necessary for the success of the prone pressure method. Gibbens,[18] Surgeon Commander of the Royal Navy, has been disappointed with the Schäfer Method and considers the Eve method superior. Hemingway,[19] after a well-conceived series of physiologic experiments on artificial respiration, concludes that more attention should be paid to the circulatory changes in assessing the value of various methods and that cardiac output, rate of oxygen uptake, and oxygen tension of venous blood are usually greater with the rocking method than with the Schäfer method.

In the rocking method the abdominal contents alternately push the diaphragm up into the chest in the head-down tilt and pull the diaphragm down with the head-up tilt, thus accomplishing respirations. Eve has also demonstrated that an artificial circulation is produced by this method with alternate filling and emptying of the heart, the backflow of blood being prevented by the valves of the heart and veins.[20] He has demonstrated mathematically that the pressure in the pulmonary artery is twice normal with rocking, thus overcoming the engorgement of the right side of the heart seen in the nearly drowned patient.[11]

The Eve method[21] consists in the rhythmical rocking of the patient through 45 degrees with a head-up and a head-down position composing one cycle. This cycle is repeated 12-15 times per minute. Eve, Mummery,[22] Gibbens,[18] and Lahiff[23] have each devised and described a simple, inexpensive, easily constructed and manipulated device similar in principle to the playground seesaw. In brief, it consists of a trestle 34 inches high (22 inches, Lahiff) with a rotary crosspiece which acts as a fulcrum. A stretcher is secured to the crosspiece. (Fig. 8.) The patient is laid face down on the

Methods of Artificial Respiration—Cont'd
Eve Rocking Method—Cont'd

stretcher, and the ankles and wrists are bound to the handles to prevent slipping. Then he is rocked up and down. The transfer takes approximately 25 seconds. Eve [24] and Gibbens[18] emphatically state that prone pressure artificial respiration be started on removal of the victim from the water and continued without interruption until rocking has begun.

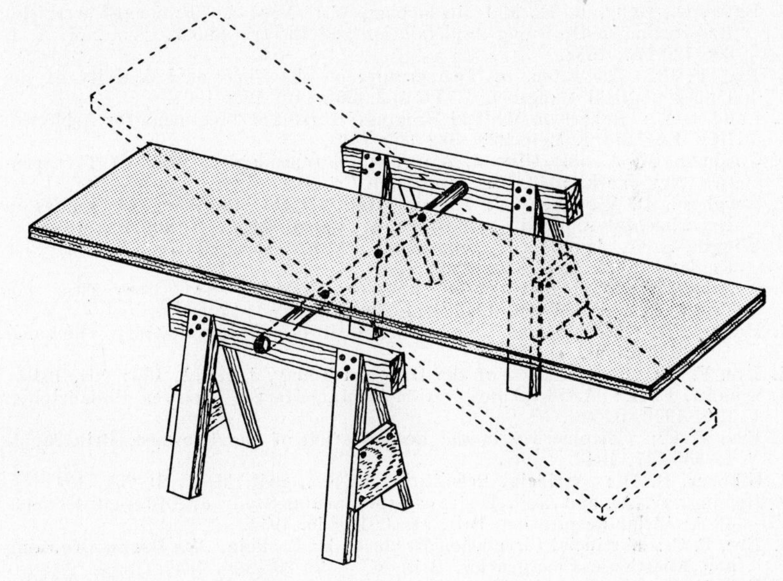

Fig. 8.—Drawing of Eve Rocking Device used in artificial respiration in drowning, showing simplicity of construction. Height of horse, 34 inches. Length of stretcher, 6 feet. Width of board wide enough to accommodate ordinary stretcher.

The manual form of this method is well suited for use in children where the patient's weight would not be too tiring. This requires two operators who stand facing each other, joining hands or jointly grasping rope quoits. The victim is laid face down on the two pairs of arms with one pair across the upper thorax and the other across the lower thighs. Then the patient is tilted up and down, 12 cycles per minute.[27] This form is advocated for rescue boats when the water is relatively calm or while waiting for the rocker to arrive.

References

1. Metropolitan Life Insurance Company: Statistical Bulletin, Water Safety Program Saves Many Lives, vol. 25, No. 6, June, 1944.
2. Metropolitan Life Insurance Company: Statistical Bulletin, Drownings Most Frequent in July, vol. 30, No. 6, June, 1949.
3. Metropolitan Life Insurance Company: Statistical Bulletin, High Toll of Civilian Drowning, vol. 24, No. 5, May, 1943.
4. Metropolitan Life Insurance Company: Statistical Bulletin, Special Hazards to Swimmers This Summer, vol. 23, No. 6, June, 1942.
5. Consolidated Edison Company of New York, Inc.: Pole Top Resuscitation, New York, 1940, 10 pp.
6. Payne, R. T.: Treatment of Drowning and Electrocution, Brit. M. J. **1**: 819-822, 1940.
7. Bates, G., Gaby, R. E., and Maclachlan, W.: Need for Prolonged Artificial Respiration in Drowning Asphyxiation and Electric Shock, Canad. M. A. J. **39**: 120-123, 1938.
8. Eve, F. C.: The Effect of Temperature on the Functional Activity of the Upper Cervical Ganglion, J. Physiol. **26**: 110, 1900-1901.
9. Lund, C. C.: Report on Medical Progress; First-Aid Treatment for Asphyxia, New England J. Med. **223**: 982-985, 1940.
10. Goodman, M. A., and Gilman, A.: The Pharmacological Basis of Therapeutics, New York, 1943, The Macmillan Co.
11. Lougheed, D. W., Janes, J. M., and Hall, G. F.: Physiological Studies in Experimental Asphyxia and Drowning, Canad. M. A. J. **40**: 423, 1939.
12. Wiggin, S. C., Saunders, P., and Small, G. A.: Resuscitation, Part 1, New England J. M. **241**: 370, 1949.
13. American National Red Cross: American National Red Cross First Aid Textbook, Philadelphia, 1945, The Blakiston Co.
14. Hughes, R. (Director and Chief of Atlantic City Beach Patrol): Personal communications.
15. Eve, F. C.: Resuscitation of the Drowned Today, J.A.M.A. **124**: 964, 1944.
16. Schafer, E. A.: Artificial Respiration in Man, Harvey Lectures, Philadelphia, 1907-1908, p. 233.
17. Eve, F. C.: Complacency in the Resuscitation of the Drowned, Brit. M. J. **1**: 535-537, 1943.
18. Gibbens, G. H.: Artificial Respiration at Sea, Brit. M. J. **2**: 751, 1942.
19. Hemingway, A., and Neil, E.: An Experimental Study of Different Methods of Artificial Respiration, Brit. M. J. **1**: 833, 1944.
20. Eve, F. C.: Artificial Circulation Produced by Rocking. Its Use in Drowning and Anesthetic Emergencies, Brit. M. J. **2**: 295-296, 1947.
21. Eve, F. C.: Lancet **29**: 95, 1932.
22. Mummery, N. H.: Resuscitation by Rocking, Brit. M. J. **1**: 759, 1943.
23. Lahiff, J. R.: Rocking Device for The Treatment of Drowning, Brit. M. J. **2**: 42, 1943.
24. Eve, F. C.: Resuscitation of the Drowned Today, Arch. Physiol. Therap. **25**: 332-337, 1944.
25. Eve, F. C.: Resuscitation Methods for Rescue Boats, Brit. M. J. **1**: 21-22, 6, 1945.

CHAPTER VII

POISONING

Introduction

Accidental poisoning in children is responsible for a large proportion of deaths yearly in the United States. It comprises about 1% of pediatric hospital admissions.

Rational emergency treatment of cases of poisoning may be effected in many instances even though the specific substance has not been identified. Nevertheless, it is most important to attempt to determine the etiologic agent in all cases of suspected poisoning. It must be emphasized that most emergency therapy is necessarily symptomatic. Nevertheless, parents or other children may know what the sick child came in contact with, swallowed, or inhaled. Contents of partially empty bottles, cans, etc., should be carefully saved and brought with the child to the doctor. Often the poisonous contents are enumerated on the label of these articles. Reference should be made to Tables I and II in the Appendix (pages 242 and 267). In addition, two other excellent reference handbooks are available for listing common poisons.[1, 2] Occasionally a TELEGRAM OR TELEPHONE CALL TO THE MANUFACTURER will give a clue to poisonous contents.

The general approach to the problem of poisoning that should be constantly kept in mind has been well stated in a recent Round Table Discussion of Pediatric Emergencies.[3]

> "The physician assumes responsibility in a poisoning case at the moment he is called, usually on the telephone. While some cases may be treated without seeing the child, it is foolish to advise emetics or other treatment if there is any chance of trouble. Delay is serious and the sooner the poison is removed from the body, the better. Parents must be advised to remove the questionable cases to the hospital immediately; there to be met by the physician. There is a medical legal side to poisoning accidents.

Introduction—Cont'd

Great care should be used in giving telephone advice because trouble may result from improper or mistaken advice."

IMMEDIATE MANAGEMENT

A. Remove the poison if possible.
B. Give antidote.
C. Administer other supportive therapy.

A. *Removal*
1. *Inhaled poisons,* especially gases.
   (A) Fresh air or oxygen.
   (B) Artificial respiration
2. *Surface poisons.*
   (A) Large amounts of water.
   (B) Soap and water.
   (C) Alcohol (for water-insoluble substances such as phenol).
   (D) Neutralize remaining poison.
      (1) If acids, use
         (a) Sodium bicarbonate.
         (b) Milk of magnesia.
         (c) Chalk.
         (d) Soap and water.
      (2) If alkalis, use
         (a) Lemon or other citrus fruit juice.
         (b) Vinegar.
3. *Surface poisons in the eye* (see page 164 et seq.).
4. *Ingested poisons.*
   (A) *Generally speaking, it is only in rare cases that emetic drugs are of any value.* Nevertheless, the household emetics listed below may frequently be used to advantage as a preliminary emergency measure. AVOID EMETICS IF STRONG ACIDS OR ALKALIS HAVE BEEN INGESTED.
      (1) *Household emetics.*

IMMEDIATE MANAGEMENT—Cont'd

A. *Removal*—Cont'd

4. *Ingested poisons*—Cont'd

(A) *Emetics*—Cont'd

(1) *Household emetics*—Cont'd

(a) Salt—2 tablespoonfuls of salt in one glass of warm water.

(b) Soapy water—¼ of glassful of a mild soapy water solution.

(c) Mustard—1 teaspoonful of dry mustard in 1 glass of warm water. Mustard is safe but not certain in its desired action. Several such doses may be administered at 15-minute intervals until vomiting is initiated.

(d) Tickle soft palate with finger.

(2) *Drugs as emetics.*

In general, most physicians are reluctant to use emetic drugs in young infants because of possible toxicity and associated central nervous system depressant action.

(a) Apomorphine hydrochloride, 1/60 gr. subcutaneously or 1/12 to 1/20 gr. orally. If vomiting does not occur with the first dose, *do not repeat dose because* in large amounts Apomorphine hydrochloride may act as a central nervous system depressant.

(b) Lavage (*TREATMENT OF CHOICE FOR REMOVING INGESTED POISONS*).*

This is generally a more efficient and certain method for removal of stomach contents. It is generally safe with two exceptions listed below. In addition to the usual lavage solutions, specific antidotes

*In addition to the recommendations listed below, refer to section on Pediatric Procedures for suggestions in performing lavage, page 208.

IMMEDIATE MANAGEMENT—Cont'd

A. *Removal*—Cont'd

4. *Ingested poisons*—Cont'd

(A) *Emetics*—Cont'd

(2) *Drugs as emetics*—Cont'd

(b) Lavage—Cont'd

as well as cathartics (when indicated) may be administered through the lavage tube. The first 200-300 c.c. of material aspirated from the stomach should be sent to a laboratory for chemical analysis for poisons.

General precautions and care during lavage.

I. Prevent aspiration into lungs.
  - (i) Turn head to side and keep head low.
  - (ii) Pinch lavage tube firmly when removing.

II. Use small amounts of liquid rather than large amounts. The liquid should be removed by suction with a large glass syringe.

Solutions generally used in lavage.

I. Water, saline, weak sodium bicarbonate.

II. Potassium permanganate 1:10,000 solution.

III. Specific and/or general antidotes.

IV. Cathartics.
  Avoid saline cathartics in phosphorus poisoning.

Contraindications to lavage.

I. Spasms of strychnine poisoning may be changed by this stimulation to fatal convulsions.

II. Erosion of esophagus due to corrosive agents such as phenol may result in perforation of the esophagus.

IMMEDIATE MANAGEMENT—Cont'd

B. *Antidotes.*

1. More specific antidotes will be enumerated below, but if the poison is unknown, the universal may be given orally following gastric lavage.

UNIVERSAL ANTIDOTE

Powdered charcoal	2 parts
Magnesium oxide	1 part
Tannic acid	1 part

Dose: 1 teaspoonful in a small glass of lukewarm water.

2. If this is not immediately available, certain simple home remedies should be utilized.
   (a) *Flour* and *starches* are particularly effective by their colloidal action on iodine.
   (b) *Strong tea,* dilute *tincture of iodine* solution (15 drops in ½ glass of water), or weak *tannic acid* are effective against alkaloids, such as atropine or morphine.
   (c) *Milk and eggs* are valuable in poisoning with heavy metals by providing protein to precipitate the poison.
   (d) General stimulants such as *strong coffee* or *tea* are valuable for ingestion of central nervous system depressants such as barbiturates or alcohol.
   (e) Oils are useful in burns from corrosives.
   (f) When acids or alkalis have been ingested, use common substances for neutralization listed under removal of surface poisons due to acids or alkalis (page 116).

3. *Antidote supplies*[1, 4, 5] (To be on hand in the Emergency Room).

Alcohol, ethyl	95%; to make 5% or 10% aqueous solution
Aminophylline, 0.24 Gm.	Several ampules for intramuscular and intravenous use
Amyl nitrite, 5 minims	Several perles
Animal charcoal	About ½ pound should be on hand at all times.

IMMEDIATE MANAGEMENT—Cont'd

B. *Antidotes*—Cont'd

3. *Antidote supplies*—Cont'd

Aromatic spirits of ammonia	Bottles and/or frangible ampules
Atropine sulfate, 0.001 Gm. (1/60 gr.)	Tablets for hypodermic use
BAL in oil	Several ampules
Caffeine sodium benzoate, 0.5 Gm. (7½ gr.)	*For intravenous use;* several ampules
Calcium gluconate, 1.375 Gm.	Several ampules of 10% solution for *intravenous* use
Carbogen (CO_2 and oxygen mixture)	
Catheters of various sizes	
Chloral hydrate, 0.3 Gm. (5 gr.)	Several tablets
Dextrose in water 50%	20 c.c. vials
Digitalis preparations for intramuscular and intravenous use	
Ephedrine sulfate, 0.05 Gm. (¾ gr.)	For oral use; Several capsules
Epinephrine 1:1000	Several 1.0 c.c. ampules
1:10,000	
1:100	Bottle for spray
Hydrochloric acid	0.5% HCl or vinegar 1:4
Magnesium oxide	Sufficient to prepare universal antidote
Magnesium sulfate	50% solution: (1) several sterile ampules, (2) several ounces
Methylene blue 1%	Several 50 c.c. ampules
Metrazol, 25% solution	Several ampules of 1 to 5 c.c.
Mouth gags	Several prepared for use
Paraldehyde	
Pentobarbital (Nembutal), 3.75 gr.	Several ampules
Pentothal Sodium, 0.12 Gm. (2 gr.)	Several ampules for *intravenous* use
Picrotoxin	20 c.c. vials (1 c.c. = 3 mg.); several ampules for *intravenous* use
Plasma, lyophilized and irradiated	
Potassium permanganate, 3 gr.	Several tablets
Prostigmine Methylsulfate 1:2000	Several ampules
1:4000	
Sodium Amytal, 0.3 Gm. (5 gr.)	Several ampules for *intravenous* use
Sodium bicarbonate	Sufficient powder for therapeutic use
Sodium chloride	Table salt or physiologic saline
Sodium formaldehyde sulfoxalate, 10 Gm.	Prepare with sterile water to make percentage solution recommended in mercurial poisoning treatment (page 129)
Sodium thiosulfate, 10%	Several 10 c.c. ampules
Starch	
Stomach tube	
Syringes	
Tannic acid	Enough powder should be on hand to prepare universal antidote

C. *Supportive therapy.*

This phase of therapy cannot be emphasized too strongly.

1. Keep the patient warm and at rest.
2. Competent medical observation and supervision are essential.

IMMEDIATE MANAGEMENT—Cont'd
C. *Supportive therapy*—Cont'd

3. Treat shock if it supervenes.
4. Use oxygen with 5% CO_2 and artificial respiration liberally in case of depressed respiration.
5. *Use all chemical antidotes, stimulants, or sedatives cautiously. Remember that the compounds formed by antidotes may be only slightly less toxic than the poison itself.*

SPECIFIC MANAGEMENT OF POISONING BY VARIOUS AGENTS

Poisoning by Ingredients Found in Household Articles

ANILINE DYES

Signs

Grayish cyanosis is outstanding feature due to methemoglobinemia.

Treatment

1. Whole blood transfusion.
2. Intravenous methylene blue, 2 mg. per kilogram of a 1% solution, should be given slowly (over a period of at least 5 minutes). If cyanosis persists for a half-hour, repeat the dose.
3. Other general supportive therapy; oxygen administration may be of value.

ANTU (Rodenticide)

Symptoms and Signs

Hypothermia, dyspnea, pleural effusion, hyperglycemia.

Treatment

1. Evacuate stomach.
2. Oxygen.

SPECIFIC MANAGEMENT OF POISONING BY VARIOUS AGENTS—Cont'd
Poisoning by Ingredients Found in Household Articles—Cont'd
ANTU (Rodenticide)—Cont'd
Treatment—Cont'd

3. Cysteine, 100 to 500 mg. per kilogram of body weight, intramuscularly.
4. Avoid parenteral fluids.

ARSENIC (Main Ingredient of Most Weed Killers)

1. Gastric lavage with soda bicarbonate solution.*
2. Force fluids.
3. Sedation and morphine for pain.
4. The latest and most specific treatment is Dimercaprol (2,3-Dimercaptropropanol) also known as British anti-lewisite or BAL. (Available in ampules from Hynson, Westcott, & Dunning, Inc., Baltimore, Md.) It is given intramuscularly as 10% solution in peanut oil. The earliest possible use of this drug is imperative. The following dosage schedule has been recommended:

BAL FOR ARSENICAL POISONING
(From Woody and Kometani: Pediatrics, 1948.[6])

	INDIVIDUAL DOSE (MG./KG.)	NUMBER OF INJECTIONS	INTERVALS (HR.)
On suspicion	2.5	3-6	4-8
Mild symptoms	2.5-3.5	6-12	4-8
Severe symptoms	3.5-5.0	6-12	4-8

5. In order to prevent reactions to BAL, administer 25 mg. ephedrine sulfate orally or intramuscularly before giving BAL.
6. Treat shock; correct fluid and electrolyte deficits.

BORIC ACID

Signs

1. "Boiled lobster" appearance of skin, particularly of face and neck.

*Recently[5a] it has been suggested that BAL be also used in lavage in cases of arsenic poisoning. The same dosage is recommended as for intramuscular use. The oily solution should be shaken with water.

2. Moderate to marked hyperpnea.
3. Abdominal tenderness.
4. Acidosis.
5. Exfoliative erythematous rash.
6. Oliguria.
7. Albuminuria.

Treatment

1. Lavage with sodium bicarbonate if taken orally.
2. Correct acidosis with sodium lactate and administer chlorides parenterally to counteract displacement by chlorides of boron in body fluids.

CAMPHOR

1. Treat as outlined under Strychnine (page 142).
2. *Oils and alcohols should be avoided because they render camphor more soluble and absorbable.*

CARBON DISULFIDE

1. Remove patient to fresh air at once.
2. Administer oxygen as soon as possible.
3. Judicious use of stimulants.
4. Supportive fluid therapy.

CARBON MONOXIDE (Illuminating Gas)

Signs

Outstanding diagnostic sign is the presence of cherry red cyanosis.

Treatment

1. Remove patient to fresh air at once.
2. Administer high concentration of oxygen.

SPECIFIC MANAGEMENT OF POISONING BY VARIOUS AGENTS—Cont'd
Poisoning by Ingredients Found in Household Articles—Cont'd
CARBON MONOXIDE (Illuminating Gas)—Cont'd
Treatment—Cont'd

3. 5 to 10% CO_2 facilitates removal by increasing respirations and decreasing pH of the blood. *This is more beneficial than oxygen alone.*
4. Artificial respiration until the patient breathes normally.
5. Keep patient warm.
6. Keep patient as quiet as possible so that the tissue demands for oxygen be kept at a minimum.
7. *Note:* Emphasis should be placed on a guarded prognosis, especially in case of coma lasting a long time.

CARBON TETRACHLORIDE

1. Immediate lavage followed by saline cathartic.
2. Calcium chloride, ¼ c.c. of a 5% solution per kilogram of body weight, or calcium gluconate, 4 to 10 c.c. of 10% solution,* given intravenously.
3. Intravenous hypertonic glucose and Hartmann's to combat acidosis and liver dysfunction.
4. Insulin, 2-3 units of U-20 to facilitate carbohydrate, fat, and protein metabolism.
5. Oxygen.
6. Transfusion.
7. No epinephrine or alcohol.
8. The administration of vitamin B_{12} may prevent liver damage.

CHLORINE GAS

1. Immediate administration of oxygen in high concentrations.
2. Relieve right heart failure and venous congestion (if present) by venesection with gradual reduction of blood volume.

---

*It is generally best to dilute solutions of calcium salts for intravenous use to a 2 to 3% solution.

3. In absence of increased venous pressure, or in presence of shock, treat with parenteral fluids to restore proper fluid volume.
4. Caffeine sodium benzoate may be used as a cardiac stimulant.
5. If acidosis is marked, treat with alkali given parenterally.
6. Inhale medicated steam or alcohol vapor.
7. Codeine may be used for severe cough.
8. Boric acid solution and ophthalmic anesthetic ointment (see page 165) for local eye discomfort.
9. Prophylactic antibiotic therapy is indicated.

CHLORDANE (Insecticide)

Symptoms

CNS irritability with convulsions.

Treatment

1. Lavage with warm water.
2. Barbiturates for restlessness or convulsions.

COCAINE (Methycaine, Butyn, Nupercaine, Tutocaine, Alypin, etc.)

A. Treatment during excitement stage.
   1. Treat as outlined under Strychnine Poisoning (page 142).

B. Treatment during stage of depression.
   1. Artificial respiration.
   2. Judicious use of respiratory stimulants.
   3. Administer oxygen.

CYANIDE

1. Prompt lavage with potassium permanganate 1:10,000 or solution of hydrogen peroxide diluted 10 times with water is indicated.

SPECIFIC MANAGEMENT OF POISONING BY VARIOUS AGENTS—Cont'd
Poisoning by Ingredients Found in Household Articles—Cont'd
CYANIDE—Cont'd

2. Sodium nitrite (0.3 to 0.5 Gm. in 10 to 15 c.c. of water) is given to produce methemoglobinemia. The methemoglobin so produced combines with the cyanide ion to form cyanmethemoglobin, which renders the cyanide ion nontoxic and nonionizable.
3. Amyl nitrite (inhalation for 30 seconds out of every 2 minutes) may be used while the sodium nitrite is being prepared.
4. Sodium thiosulfate (50 c.c. of a 50% solution intravenously) is then slowly injected in order to convert the cyanide released by dissociation of cyanmethemoglobin to thiocyanate.
5. Oxygen.
6. Blood transfusions.
7. Sometimes the intravenous administration of a 1% methylene blue solution is used to form methemoglobin.
8. Cytochrome C and sodium succinate have been found to be of value experimentally. Thus, they may be used if all other methods fail. If available, cytochrome C in doses of 25-50 mg. may be used for the anoxia. Sodium succinate may also be used in doses of 3 to 5 c.c. of a 30% solution intravenously at a rate of 1 c.c. per second. It may be necessary to use 40 to 60 c.c.

DDT

1. Gastric lavage with warm water.
2. Intravenous calcium gluconate, 5 to 10 c.c. of a 10% solution.
3. Atropine and barbiturates to counteract convulsions as outlined under Strychnine Poisoning (page 142).
4. Therapeutic doses of Dilantin Sodium may be necessary to control convulsions.
5. High protein diet.

6. Ensure adequate fluid intake.
7. Glucose should be administered orally or parenterally.

ETHYLENE GLYCOL—For symptoms and treatment, see Oxalate Poisoning (page 131).

FLUORIDES (Including Hydrofluoric Acid)[6a]

A. Initial home treatment.
   1. Large quantities of milk orally.

B. Hospital treatment.[7]
   1. Gastric lavage with lime water (15% calcium hydroxide).
   2. Lime water orally every half hour.
   3. Liberal oral use of an amphoteric antacid, such as Amphojel. (A recent discussion[8] of the toxicity of sodium fluoride in man indicates that the administration of sodium fluoride alone causes gastritis and regurgitation because of the formation of hydrofluoric acid in the stomach. Minimal gastrointestinal disturbances are said to be effected by the administration of amphoteric antacid).
   4. Intravenous calcium gluconate (5 to 10 c.c. of a 10% solution) at first sign of tetany or hypocalcemia.
   5. Intravenous dextrose and saline in accordance with body weight needs.
   6. External burns may be prevented by frequently washing the skin soiled by vomitus and/or excretions.

FORMALDEHYDE

1. Lavage with dilute ammonia water (0.2 per cent) or egg albumin water.
2. Fluids, Hartmann's solution.
3. Plasma or blood.
4. Respiratory stimulants.

HYDROCARBONS (Especially Kerosene)

Symptoms and Signs

1. Vomiting, gagging, choking, and coughing.
2. Drowsiness.
3. Kerosene odor to breath or vomitus.

Treatment

1. Lavage early (if large amounts have been swallowed only) with warm water or weak sodium bicarbonate solution.

   USE CARE TO AVOID ASPIRATION OF THE OILS. *AVOID EMETICS!*
2. Leave 30 to 60 c.c. of mineral or olive oil in the stomach.
3. Oxygen should be used for hyperpnea.
4. Transfusions of whole blood.
5. Penicillin in therapeutic doses to control or prevent infection.
6. Cold packs and adequate hydration to control hyperpyrexia.
7. Digitalize if congestive heart failure is imminent.

IODINE

1. Lavage with soluble starch solution, sodium thiosulfate (5%), or egg white. Continue lavage until all traces of iodine are removed.
2. Intravenous fluids, especially isotonic saline.
3. Treat shock if present.

LEAD

1. Gastric lavage.
2. Saline cathartics.
3. Fluids intravenously.
4. In acute lead poisoning, a high calcium diet is used to bring about lead deposition in the bones. In lead colic,

SPECIFIC MANAGEMENT OF POISONING BY VARIOUS AGENTS—Cont'd
Poisoning by Ingredients Found in Household Articles—Cont'd
LEAD—Cont'd
4. Acute lead poisoning—Cont'd

the intravenous injection of 15 c.c. of a 5% solution of calcium chloride is often followed by immediate disappearance of the pain.

LYE (Also in Cases of AMMONIA POISONING)

1. An antidote is of no value unless administered within a few minutes following ingestion. Lavage with dilute vinegar, lemon juice, or weak acids.
2. Follow by several ounces of olive oil or flour paste.
3. If an hour or more has elapsed, avoid lavage and only aspirate secretions from pharynx.
4. Olive oil orally frequently in small amounts.
5. Give a sedative-analgesic. Codeine is usually helpful.
6. A string may be swallowed and left in place to aid in case of stricture.
7. Dilatations with a soft rubber eyeless catheter filled with mercury or lead shot should be started on the fourth day.[9]

MERCURY (Especially as Bichloride Tablets or Solution)

1. Immediate and repeated lavage with raw white of egg or milk is necessary to precipitate the metal.
2. 5 to 10% solution of sodium formaldehyde sulfoxalate freshly made is excellent for lavage. About 250 c.c. should be used for lavage and 100 to 200 c.c. left in the stomach.
3. Sodium hyposulfite, chalk, milk of magnesia, and starch paste is excellent for lavage.
4. Gastric lavage twice a day with 4% sodium bicarbonate.
5. Colonic irrigation with several hundred cubic centimeters of 2% sodium acetate.
6. Maintain body fluids; isotonic saline or Ringer's solution in amounts depending on the age of the child should

be given parenterally. This aids in diuresis and protects the kidney from high concentrations of mercury. Continue unless edema or oliguria develops.

7. The most specific treatment available is with Dimercaprol or BAL (10% in oil), dosage schedule and precautions as outlined in section on Arsenic Poisoning (page 122).

METHYL ALCOHOL

1. Gastric lavage with 3 to 5% sodium bicarbonate.
2. Hartmann's solution for acidosis (very important) intravenously. (The CO_2 combining power should be checked frequently.)
3. Oxygen.
4. Respiratory stimulants. (Caffeine sodium benzoate.)
5. Artificial respiration.
6. Plasma for shock.

NAPHTHALENE (Moth Balls)

1. Copious lavage with water.
2. AVOID OILS, especially castor oil, because moth balls are soluble in oil.

NICOTINE

1. Lavage with tannic acid, strong tea or coffee, or potassium permanganate solution 1:10,000.
2. Artificial respiration to be continued as long as necessary.
3. Oxygen.
4. Respiratory stimulants are of some value if respiratory depression is present.

SPECIFIC MANAGEMENT OF POISONING BY VARIOUS AGENTS—Cont'd
Poisoning by Ingredients Found in Household Articles—Cont'd

NITRATES (Due to Well Water with High Nitrate Content or Bismuth Subnitrate)

1. *Severe cases*

   Methylene blue, 1-2 mg. per kilogram of body weight, intravenously, given as 1% solution.*

2. *Mild cases*

   Methylene blue, 65-100 mg. per kilogram orally.

OXALATES AND OXALIC ACID (In Bleaching Powders)

1. Lavage with 0.1% potassium permanganate followed by 5% calcium chloride, chalk, or lime solution.
2. Calcium gluconate (2 to 10 c.c. of 10% solution) or 5% solution of calcium chloride (¼ c.c. per kilogram) may be given intravenously if tetany occurs.

PHENOL (Cresol, Creosote, Lysol)

As first aid, give olive oil, cod liver oil, egg white.

1. Remove as much of the drug as possible quickly.
2. Lavage with olive oil or glycerine 10% provides a solvent for phenol.
3. Do not use alcohol or mineral oil, as alcohol facilitates absorption and mineral oil is a poor solvent.
4. Leave several ounces of olive oil in the stomach after lavage.
5. Force parenteral fluids to protect kidneys.
6. Castor oil or 50% alcohol should be used to remove phenol from superficial areas such as skin and mucous membranes.

---

*Available through Wm. H. Rorer, Inc., 254 South Fourth Street, Philadelphia, Pa.

SPECIFIC MANAGEMENT OF POISONING BY VARIOUS AGENTS—Cont'd
Poisoning by Ingredients Found in Household Articles—Cont'd

PHOSPHORUS

1. Gastric lavage with
   (a) 0.2% copper sulfate solution, or
   (b) potassium permanganate solution 1:1000, or
   (c) 2% hydrogen peroxide solution.
2. *Do not give a cathartic.*
3. Introduce 50 to 100 c.c. of liquid petrolatum into stomach.
4. Treat dehydration, acidosis, and shock.
5. Catheterize bladder as needed.
6. If there is any question of concurrent poisoning, use BAL.
7. Treat local phosphorus burns with 1% copper sulfate solution and bland topical ointments.
8. The attending physician should protect himself from vomitus during lavage of patient.

POTASSIUM BROMATE[10, 11]

1. Emetic.
   (a) Teaspoonful of mustard powder in glassful of warm (not hot) water, or
   (b) Zinc sulfate, ½ teaspoonful in water, followed by copious drinking of water, or
   (c) Apomorphine, 5 mg. intramuscularly, and/or
   (d) Wash out stomach with stomach tube.
2. Sodium thiosulfate (Hypo), 1 level teaspoonful in water. This may precede but should always follow the emetic.
3. Demulcent drinks such as milk, flour, and water, cereal gruel.
4. If shock is present, treat for shock, but avoid central nerous system stimulants.
5. For pain (gastritis), give morphine, subcutaneously. Dose for children, 5 mg. or more depending on age and weight.

6. Sodium thiosulfate solution, 1%, intravenously by drip, 100 to 500 c.c. If not feasible, give 10 to 50 c.c. of a 10% solution.

Note: The physician should be requested to have the vomitus or gastric washings analyzed for the presence of bromine (as such, or as bromide and bromate). The urine should also be tested for the presence of bromide in order to establish the diagnosis.

POTASSIUM CHLORATE AND PERCHLORATE

1. Lavage with copious amounts of warm water.
2. Saline catharsis.
3. Parenteral fluids to induce diuresis.
4. Transfusion and oxygen plus other supportive therapy.
5. Treat methemoglobinemia if it develops with methylene blue, as outlined under Nitrite Poisoning (page 131).

PYRETHRUM (AND ROTENONE)

1. Copious lavage with water.
2. General supportive therapy.
3. Institute treatment as outlined under Nicotine Poisoning (page 130).

SILVER

Lavage with sodium chloride solution.
Treat as under Mercury Poisoning (page 129).

SODIUM HYPOSULFITE (Clorox)

Signs

1. Vomiting.

SPECIFIC MANAGEMENT OF POISONING BY VARIOUS AGENTS—Cont'd
Poisoning by Ingredients Found in Household Articles—Cont'd
SODIUM HYPOSULFITE (Clorox)—Cont'd
Signs—Cont'd

2. Corrosive burns of chin, lips, tongue, pharynx, and larynx.
3. Aphonia.

Treatment

1. Lavage with copious amounts of warm water or weak acids.
2. Apply emollients to the accessible areas.
3. General supportive therapy.

THALLIUM

1. Lavage with sodium thiosulfite.
2. Administer 20 c.c. of 3% sodium thiosulfite intravenously.
3. Treat shock if present.
4. Use BAL as outlined under section on Arsenic Poisoning (page 122).

TURPENTINE

1. Lavage with copious amounts of warm water or weak sodium bicarbonate solution.
2. Saline catharsis.
3. General supportive therapy.

Poisoning Due to Drugs*

ANTIMONY—Symptomatology and treatment as outlined under **ARSENIC** (page 122)

ATROPINE (Belladonna, Scopolamine, Homatropine)

1. Gastric lavage with dilute tincture of iodine, strong tea, or 4% tannic acid solution if child has consumed large amounts.

---

*See addendum for following: Aconite, page 236; Aminophylline, page 236; Carbon Monoxide Poisoning, page 236; Dichloricide and Dichlorphenol, page 236; Ethyl Alcohol, page 236; Fluoroacetate (Compound 1080), page 237; Iron, page 237; Magnesium Sulfate, page 237; Methyl Alcohol, page 238; Phosphoric Acid Esters (Thiophos, T.E.P., and Related Insecticides), page 238; Salicylate Intoxication, page 238; Zinc Stearate, page 238.

2. In the stage of excitement a short-acting barbiturate such as Seconal, ½ gr. to 1½ gr., may be used. Prolonged use and large doses must be avoided because of the secondary stage of depression and respiratory paralysis.
3. In the stage of depression, one or more of the following stimulants may be used:
   Caffeine sodium benzoate, 1 to 5 gr., depending upon the age and weight
   Ephedrine sulfate, 8 to 48 mg. (⅛ to ¾ gr.)
   Strychnine sulfate, 0.3 to 0.6 mg. (1/200 to 1/100 gr.)
   Picrotoxin—See Barbiturate Poisoning (page 135)
4. In respiratory paralysis, artificial respiration.
5. Fever may be effectively controlled by sponging, ice packs, and parenteral fluids.
6. Pilocarpine, 5 mg. repeated at intervals until mouth is moist. This merely adds to the patient's comfort and relieves visual symptoms to some extent.

BARBITURATES*

1. Establish an adequate airway.
2. Give artificial respiration as needed.
3. Oxygen through the airway at 6 liters per minute.
4. Gastric lavage with warm water or 1:2000 potassium permanganate solution to remove unabsorbed poison still remaining in the stomach.
5. Use of analeptics.
   (a) *Picrotoxin,* 3 to 6 mg. intramuscularly (1/20 to 3/32 gr.) every 30 minutes until corneal or swallowing reflexes appear. When reflexes appear, continue Picrotoxin in doses of 3 to 6 mg. intramuscularly as needed to maintain the reflexes. IT IS IMPOR-

*More deaths were caused in 1947 by accidental poisoning in children by barbiturates than by any other drugs (Mortality Statistics, Metropolitan Life Insurance Co.

SPECIFIC MANAGEMENT OF POISONING BY VARIOUS AGENTS—Cont'd
Poisoning Due to Drugs—Cont'd
BARBITURATES—Cont'd

TANT TO REALIZE THAT THE RESPONSE TO PICROTOXIN IS SLOWER WHEN LONG-ACTING BARBITURATES ARE INVOLVED IN THE POISONING THAN WHEN THE SHORT-ACTING ONES ARE INVOLVED. EXERCISE CAUTION. IF AN UNTOWARD REACTION SUCH AS TWITCHES OR CONVULSIONS OCCURS, AN INTRAVENOUS BARBITURATE SUCH AS PENTOTHAL SODIUM MAY BE USED IN SMALL DOSES TO COUNTERACT THE UNTOWARD REACTION.

(b) *Amphetamine (Benzedrine) sulfate* may also be used to treat barbiturate poisoning. It is prepared as 10 mg. in 1 c.c. of isotonic sodium chloride for intravenous use. 10 mg. are given at once and then 10 mg. every half hour until reflexes are present or the patient reacts.

(c) *Metrazol*,[12] 0.5 c.c. of a 10% solution, should be administered intravenously as an orientation dose. Mild cases will usually respond. However, if this dose does not cause visible changes in the patient, it should be repeated every 15 minutes until the patient responds adequately.

6. Use of ephedrine sulfate[13] in doses of 10 to 30 mg. intramuscularly repeated every hour or two as needed. The use of this drug, of course, elevates the blood pressure and acts also as a respiratory stimulant.
7. Intravenous fluids including sufficient vitamins. Avoid excess sodium administration.
8. Prophylactic chemotherapy and antibiotic therapy (pneumonia is frequently an important contributing cause of death in these patients).
9. Judicious use of diuretic agents in the presence of edema.

10. Proper, careful nursing care is most essential.
11. Saline cathartic may be beneficial.

BENADRYL (and Other Antihistaminic Agents)

Experimental and clinical evidence indicates that infants and children generally respond to toxic amounts of antihistaminics with marked CNS irritation resulting in convulsions and hyperthermia. It has been stated[14] that barbiturates are contraindicated in convulsions due to toxic amounts of antihistaminics in children. Sufficient experimental evidence is available, however, to indicate that barbiturates should be used.[14a] The problems encountered in therapy may be summarized:

1. Short-acting barbiturates (Pentothal Sodium, Sodium Seconal or even Pentobarbital Sodium) should be given in small, fractional doses; 1 c.c. per minute of a 2.5% solution intravenously.
2. Strict attention must be directed toward observing secondary respiratory depression (usually resulting from too much or too rapid administration of barbiturates). Should this develop, Metrazol should be administered in small quantities as listed on page 136 under Barbiturate Poisoning.

Actually, Seevers[14a] has stated ". . . treatment represents a fine quantitative assessment of the relative irritability of the CNS system and the titration of this irritability with the appropriate drug, whether it be a stimulant or a depressant."

3. If hyperthermia exists, use
   (a) Cooling sponges.
   (b) Cooling enemas.
   (c) Ice packs

BENZEDRINE (and Dexedrine)

1. Lavage stomach with copious amounts of warm water.
2. If marked CNS stimulation is present, use barbiturates as outlined in section on treatment of Convulsions (page 41).
3. If coma is present, symptomatic and supportive therapy is indicated only. Barbiturates, in this stage, are definitely contraindicated.

BENZENE DERIVATIVES (Acetanilid, Aniline, Nitrobenzene, Aminopyrine, and Antipyrine)

1. Gastric lavage.
2. Saline catharsis.
3. Intravenous methylene blue as outlined in section on Nitrate Poisoning (page 131).
4. Artificial respiration.
5. Oxygen.
6. Transfusions.
7. Other measures listed under Barbiturate Poisoning (page 135).

BISMUTH SUBNITRATE—See treatment of **NITRATE POISONING** (page 131)

CHLORAL HYDRATE

1. Gastric lavage with warm water.
2. External heat to maintain body temperature.
3. Oxygen.
4. Respiratory stimulants as needed for respiratory depression.
5. 10% dextrose in water intravenously in accordance with body weight needs.
6. Ephedrine sulfate, 25 mg. intramuscularly, to elevate blood pressure.

CURARE

The increase in use of this drug and its derivatives in the treatment of spastic states as seen in poliomylelitis and spastic paraplegias warrants its inclusion here.

1. Prostigmine Methylsulfate, 1.0 c.c. of a 1:4000 solution intravenously.
2. Continuous artificial respiration until patient can breathe normally.
3. Oxygen.

DIGITALIS

1. Gastric lavage if poisoning is due to large oral intake.
2. If due to continued overdosage, give moderate fluids.
3. Oxygen.
4. If severe ventricular tachycardia results, treat as on page 22.

EPHEDRINE

1. Gastric lavage.
2. Sedation with barbiturates.
3. General supportive therapy.

IRON[15] (In the Form of Ferrous Sulfate Present in Hematinic Tablets and Elixirs)

1. Prompt lavage with copious amounts of warm water is indicated.
2. Administer milk and egg white either orally or by gavage.
3. Sodium carbonate may be helpful if given early in amounts equal to the amount of iron ingested. Do not use BAL.

MECHOLYL (Also Pilocarpine, Arecoline, and Muscarine)

1. Atropine sulfate, 0.25 to 0.6 mg. intravenously ($\frac{1}{250}$ to $\frac{1}{100}$ gr.).

2. Respiratory stimulants.
3. If an asthmatic attack is precipitated, epinephrine in usual doses is indicated.
4. Plasma for shock.

NITRITES (Bismuth Subnitrate, Amylnitrite, Sodium Nitrite, or Spirits of Glyceryl Trinitrate)

1. Gastric lavage with warm water.
2. Saline catharsis.
3. If syncope occurs, ephedrine in usual doses may be of value.
4. Oxygen.
5. Transfusions.
6. Methylene blue in presence of methemoglobinemia. (See section on Nitrates, page 131.)

OPIATES AND MORPHINE

1. Repeated lavage with water.
2. Leave 4 to 5 ounces of a 1:10,000 solution of potassium permanganate in the stomach.
3. Respiratory and central nervous system stimulants.
4. Oxygen.
5. External heat.
6. Artificial respiration.

POTASSIUM

1. 15 to 25 c.c. of 10% calcium gluconate intravenously to counteract potassium inhibition of heart. This should be given slowly and diluted with distilled water to a 2% concentration.
2. 150-250 c.c. of hypertonic glucose solution to act as diuretic and to enhance deposition of glycogen in liver.

3. Oxygen.
4. Repeated EKG examinations should be requested to determine recovery from heart block.

PHENOLPHTHALEIN (As in Analaz, Ex-Lax, Phenolax, and Cathartic Chewing Gums)

1. Repeated lavage.
2. Diagnosis may be confirmed by the development of a pink color on the addition of alkali to the lavaged material. stool, or water.

QUININE

1. Lavage with 1:1000 potassium permanganate.
2. Saline catharsis.
3. Intravenous fluids.
4. Stimulants as indicated.

SALICYLATES (Methyl Salicylate, Salicylic Acid, and Salicylates)

1. Gastric lavage with water or 1:1000 permanganate of potassium.
2. Early, give sodium chloride intravenously; later correct the ketosis as it develops. It should be emphasized that no attempt should be made to administer alkali unless the CO_2 combining power and blood pH are determined. It is clear that the administration of alkali during the early phases of respiratory alkalosis would be detrimental, whereas it would be useful during the later phase of true metabolic acidosis.
3. Glucose solution intravenously.
4. Sedatives to control excitability and hyperpnea.
5. Avoid all types of stimuli.

STRYCHNINE

(Causes more than 1/3 of all deaths from poisoning in children.)

1. Lavage should not be done during convulsive attacks.
2. Give large doses of short-acting barbiturates intravenously and repeat if necessary to stop convulsions but not to depress respirations or blood pressure. For practical purposes the fractional method outlined in the Treatment of Tetanus (page 48) may be used.
3. Lavage as soon as patient is asleep with 1:1000 potassium permanganate; tincture of iodine, 1:250; 2% tannic acid, or strong tea.
4. Activated charcoal which absorbs strychnine should be placed in the stomach through the lavage tube.
5. Ether may be used temporarily to control convulsions.
6. Avoid all types of stimuli.
7. Catheterize bladder to ensure continuous evacuation of bladder and thus prevent reabsorption of strychnine from urine in the bladder.

TRIDIONE

1. Gastric lavage.
2. If patient is comatose, treat as outlined under Barbiturate Poisoning (page 135).

ZINC (Zinc Chloride or Zinc Sulfate)

1. If ingested orally, lavage followed by catharsis.
2. If zinc stearate powder is ingested, aspirate secretions, give oxygen or oxygen-helium.

SPECIFIC MANAGEMENT OF POISONING BY VARIOUS AGENTS—Cont'd

Food Poisoning

MUSHROOMS

1. Lavage.
2. Saline catharsis.
3. Fluids—glucose, plasma, blood.
4. If of muscarine type, give atropine sulfate, 1/250 to 1/100 gr.

JIMSON WEED (Stinkweed, Thorn Apple)—Stramonium Poisoning (See under **ATROPINE**, page 133)

BOTULISM

The severe type of botulism occasionally seen requires prompt treatment. The symptoms which may be present (which must be differentiated from those seen in acute bulbar poliomyelitis) are listed:

1. Abdominal pain.
2. Vomiting.
3. Difficulty in breathing.
4. Double vision.
5. Flaccid musculature, especially neck and extremities.

Treatment

1. Administration of botulinus antitoxin; 5,000 to 10,000 units of polyvalent antitoxin should be given intravenously after proper sensitivity testing.
2. Parenteral fluid therapy.
3. Prophylactic antibiotics.

References

1. Brooks, V. J., and Alyea, H. N.: Poisons: Their Chemical Identification and Emergency Treatment, New York, 1946, D. Van Nostrand Co., Inc.
2. Frear, D. E. H., et al.: Pest Control Materials, Maine Agric. Exp. Stat. Misc. Publ. No. 613, 1949.
3. Aikman, J.: Round Table Discussion on Pediatric Medical Emergencies, Pediatrics 2: 209, 1948.

4. Chittenden, R. F., and Mapes, R.: Accidental Poisoning in Children, California & West. Med. **56**: 137, 1942.
5. Hyman, H. T.: An Integrated Practice of Medicine, Philadelphia, 1947, W. B. Saunders Co.
5a. Gold, H.: Household Poisoning. II. In Conference on Therapy, American Journal of Medicine **7**: 374, March, 1950.
6. Woody, N. C., and Kometani, J. T.: BAL in the Treatment of Arsenic Ingestion in Children, Pediatrics **1**: 372, 1948.
6a. Shurts, J. J.: Hydrofluoric Acid Poisoning, J.A.M.A. **140**: 658, 1949.
7. Peters, J. H.: Use of Calcium Orally and Parenterally in Poisoning With Fluorides, Am. J. M. Sc. **216**: 278, 1948.
8. Black, M. M., et al.: The Toxicity of Sodium Fluoride in Man, New York State J. Med. **49**: 1187, 1949.
8a. Rubin, M. B., et al.: Ingestion of Poisons in Children: A Survey of 250 Admissions to Children's Hospital, Clin. Proc. Child. Hosp. Wash. (D. C.) **5**: 57, 1949.
9. Kernodle, G. W., et al.: Lye Poisoning in Children, Am. J. Dis. Child. **75**: 135, 1948.
10. Thompson, H. C., and Westfall, S. W.: Potassium Bromate Poisoning: Report of a Case Due to Ingestion of a "Cold Wave" Neutralizer, J. Pediat. **34**: 362, 1949.
11. Brunner, M. J. (Dermatologic Consultant, The Toni Co.): Personal communication.
12. Koppanyi, T.: Metrazol in Barbiturate Poisoning. In reference 8a.
13. Goodman, L., and Gilman, A.: The Pharmacologic Basis of Therapeutics, New York, 1941, The Macmillan Co., p. 143.
14. David, J. H., and Hunt, H. H.: Accidental Benadryl Poisoning: Report of a Fatal Case, J. Pediat. **34**: 358, 1949.
14a. Seevers, M. H.: Personal communication.
15. Nelson, W. E.: Iron Poisoning, J. Pediat. **36**: 397, 1950.

CHAPTER VIII

CARE OF THE PREMATURE INFANT

Introduction

The birth and care of a premature infant represents an emergency which requires not only knowledge concerning the management of the infant, but also knowledge of the underlying physiologic mechanisms and handicaps peculiar to the premature, which may precipitate other emergency conditions. It is for this reason that this detailed section on the premature baby is presented.

A premature infant is one who weighs 2,500 grams (5½ pounds) or less at birth. Premature infants ordinarily constitute 5 to 8 % of all live births but are responsible for over 50% of neonatal deaths. The mortality rate is inversely proportional to the birth weight. Under good care, the prognosis for survival for varying weight groups of premature infants is generally in accordance with the following percentages:

Less than 1,000 grams	About 10%
1,000 to 1,500 grams	About 40-50%
1,501 to 2,000 grams	About 78%
2,001 to 2,500 grams	About 95%

Premature infants suffer from a number of anatomic and physiologic handicaps due to immaturity of various systems not fully prepared to function until term. The lower the birth weight, the greater is the immaturity. The following functions are particularly handicapped in premature infants, the degree varying with the degree of prematurity: respiration, circulation, body temperature regulation, digestion, renal function, and liver function. In addition, there is increased susceptibility to infection, increased tendency to birth injury, increased capillary fragility, inadequate antenatal storage of minerals, vitamins, and immune substances, and incomplete development of enzyme systems. The following

Introduction—Cont'd

disturbances, more commonly seen in premature infants, should be kept in mind as possible complications in premature management: anoxia, congenital atelectasis, intracranial hemorrhage, pneumonia, diarrhea, infections, acidosis, edema, anemia, congenital malformations and retrolental fibroplasia (the latter particularly noted in small premature infants).

Emergency care of the premature infant should actually go back to before birth. Anoxia is one of the great hazards for the premature infant during labor and delivery and at the time of birth. According to Clifford,[1] when obstetric conditions permit, the method of delivery most likely to produce a vigorous, active, premature infant in good condition is delivery from below by episiotomy and low forceps without administration of any kind of analgesic or anesthetic to the mother. If an anesthetic is used during delivery, it should be caudal, spinal, or local infiltration anesthesia. Gentle fundal pressure is preferred by some obstetricians to the use of low forceps. Vitamin K should be administered to all women as soon as labor starts.

From a prophylactic point of view, cooperation by the obstetric department in certain phases of the management of premature labor is essential to give the premature infant its maximum chance to survive. The following recommendations* might well be prominently posted in the delivery room and on the obstetric wards as guides for the management of premature labor:

1. In case of rupture of membranes before the thirty-sixth week of pregnancy, no effort should be made to induce labor. Bed rest should be provided, and the administration of a suitable antibiotic is desirable. Instruction should be given in proper perineal hygiene. Labor may not ensue for 5, 10, or 40 days. Each day of additional

*From a set of instructions for the premature by The Departments of Obstetrics and Gynecology and Pediatrics of the University of Colorado Medical Center.

Introduction—Cont'd

intrauterine life improves the prognosis for the unborn infant.

2. The mother should have no analgesia during labor. The premature baby's respiratory center cannot recover from these analgesic agents as well as that of a full-term infant.
3. If anesthesia is necessary, use local anesthesia or low spinal anesthesia for delivery. Never use an intravenous or inhalation anesthetic. The premature baby's survival is handicapped by any type of general anesthesia.
4. A competent person should be available in the delivery room to take over the care of the newborn, so that the obstetrician can give his undivided attention to the mother. This person can devote his attention to establishing normal extrauterine breathing and to preserving the body temperature of the newborn.
5. An episiotomy should be done in most cases to protect the baby's head from the obstructing perineal body.
6. Elective low forceps are to be done if there is any delay in the perineal stage of labor. Never apply forceps on a premature head at a higher level than the outlet.
7. Vitamin K should be given to the mother during labor and to the baby soon after it is born.

Conditions at birth and in the first 24 hours are especially hazardous. Over one-half of premature deaths take place on the first day. Immediate care and a scientific and systematic plan of management for the newborn premature infant constitutes an emergency. The chances for the survival for the premature infant are greatly increased by expert hospital care.

1. The delivery room should be warm, 72 to 75 degrees Fahrenheit.
2. To conserve the infant's body heat, a sterile blanket that has been warmed should be ready for the reception of the infant.

Introduction—Cont'd

3. Suitable apparatus for suction of mouth and upper respiratory tract, including a laryngoscope and catheter for tracheal aspiration, should be provided. Oxygen tank with mechanism for measuring and controlling the amount and pressure of gas and a suitable mask for the infant should be available. With delivery of the baby, air passages are cleared by postural drainage and suction of the mouth, nose, and pharynx. If infant should fail to breathe spontaneously, some type of resuscitation is necessary (see Section on Resuscitation of the Newborn, page 97). There is considerable danger in applying rhythmic hand pressure to the chest and this should not be done. Stimulants are of questionable value.
4. The cord should not be clamped until pulsation has ceased so that the infant may receive the full complement of placental blood.
5. The infant is transferred to an incubator which has been warmed. Incubators are indispensable for the care of premature infants. An incubator must supply heat, oxygen, and humidity. It also provides isolation. There must be freedom from fire hazard, and the infant should be visible. Of additional practical importance is the ease with which the baby may be handled within the incubator. The Gordon-Armstrong incubator meets these qualifications, is easy to operate, and is relatively inexpensive. For the very small premature infants, the Isolette Incubator has certain advantages.
6. An immediate appraisal[2] of the infant's general condition should be made to determine:
   (a) Adequacy of respiration.
   (b) Any evidence of serious congenital anomalies.
   (c) Evidence of jaundice, hemorrhage, or skin eruption.
7. The premature infant is then ready to be transported to the nursery in the incubator. Here, further evaluation[2] of the infant can be made, including:

Introduction—Cont'd

(a) Review mother's prenatal, labor, and delivery history.
(b) Estimate degree of prematurity of the infant.
(c) Further examination of the infant.

If satisfactory hospital care is not available, the premature infant should be transferred via ambulance, in the incubator with oxygen and temperature regulated, to a nearby premature center, if the infant's condition permits.

Care in the Nursery

1. All premature infants should be given oxygen for 48 hours because of the tendency to develop anoxia. Anoxemia may be present in the absence of visible cyanosis and can in itself further depress respiratory control. A 3- to 4-pound premature infant may be kept in an atmosphere of 50 to 60% oxygen for days, and in the case of a 2- to 3-pound premature infant, the period may be for weeks.
2. Maintenance of optimal body temperature. A temperature of about 97 degrees Fahrenheit is a satisfactory normal temperature. The premature infant's temperature should be taken by axilla for 3 minutes. Because of the paucity of subcutaneous fat, axillary temperature is an adequate index of body temperature. The temperature of the baby and the incubator should be taken and recorded every 3 hours. As a starting point, the incubator temperature should be about 90 degrees Fahrenheit for the 2- to 3-pound infant, 85 degrees for the 3- to 4-pound infant, and 80 degrees for the 4- to 5-pound infant with variation from these figures as indicated by the baby's body temperature.
3. The baby's position should be changed every 3 hours. This 3-hour interval will coincide with his time of feeding and taking temperature so that a minimal amount

Care in Nursery—Cont'd

3. Change of position—Cont'd

of handling of the premature infant is done. Change of position facilitates lung expansion, which for premature infants may not be complete up to 3 or 4 weeks. For this reason the baby should not be overclothed, to allow greater freedom of movement. This also permits better muscular development.

4. Aseptic technique. This includes the use of gowns and masks. The hands should be thoroughly washed with soap and water between handling of babies, particularly before feeding and after diapering. Personnel with any evidence of skin, respiratory, or gastrointestinal infection should be excluded from the nursery.
5. *Care of the skin.* To prevent trauma of the skin and excessive handling, it is advisable that no bath shall be given and that no antiseptic ointments be used. After stool, the diaper area may be gently cleansed with sterile mineral oil.
6. *Feeding.* Nothing is given by mouth for the first 12 to 24 to 48 hours, depending on the size and condition of the premature infant. Should there be evidence of edema, this initial starvation period should be further prolonged. Then, 5% glucose every 3 hours is given for a period of 12 to 24 hours. Following this, a well-diluted milk mixture is started. Initial feedings of either glucose solution or milk mixture are small, 2 to 4 c.c. to 4 to 8 c.c. or more, depending on the size of the premature infant. Caloric and fluid requirements are low in the early days of life. The amount of each feeding and the concentration of the feeding mixture is gradually increased to give, by about the end of the first week, 120 calories per kilogram and 150 c.c. per kilogram if a high protein, low fat milk mixture with added carbohydrate, such as Alacta formula, is used.* This type of formula

*Several proprietary products which meet these requirements are available. Among them are Alacta and Dryco.

Care in Nursery—Cont'd
6. *Feeding*—Cont'd

is of particular value for the smaller premature infants. Larger premature infants do well on breast milk or on evaporated milk formulas. Alacta is a powdered milk prepared from equal parts of skimmed milk and whole milk. Alacta formula is high in protein, high in carbohydrate, high in minerals, and low in fats. Table VIII illustrates a method of meeting the requirements of an infant weighing 1500 grams by a gradually increasing food intake. A schedule such as this is to be used as a base from which one individualizes the feeding of each infant according to his ability to ingest and retain the amounts offered. The proportion of the feeding mixture is:

Alacta, 1 tablespoonful
Dextri-Maltose #2, 5 grams
Water, 2¼ ounces

Fluid requirements are attained by the third day and maintenance caloric requirements by the fifth day. By the eighth day, this mixture in the amounts indicated in Table VIII gives adequate fluid and calories for growth.

TABLE VIII. INITIAL FEEDINGS EVERY THREE HOURS FOR INFANT WEIGHING 1,500 GRAMS

(From Gordon: Prematurity. In Advances in Pediatrics, 1947.[3])

AGE	5 PER CENT GLUCOSE (C.C./FEEDING)	FEEDING MIXTURE (C.C./FEEDING)	TOTAL FLUID (C.C./KG./ 24 HOURS)	TOTAL CALORIES PER KG./24 HR.
0-12 hr.	0	0		
12-24 hr.	8	0	20	--
24-36 hr.	8	4		
36-48 hr.	8	8	75	30
	Water			
3, 4, 5 days	8	12-16	105-135	50-70
6, 7 days	5	20-25	135-160	85-105
8 days	0	30	160	125

Care in Nursery—Cont'd
6. *Feeding*—Cont'd

The usual feeding interval is every 3 hours. The method of feeding depends on the vigor of the infant and his ability to suck and swallow. The smaller and weaker premature infant has a weak swallowing and sucking reflex and should be gavaged every 3 hours. When the infant sucks vigorously on the catheter, a medicine dropper with rubber tip may be used or a Brecht feeder (without the bulb). These feeding methods are to be carried out in the incubator. Bottle feeding may be given when the infant becomes more vigorous. Vitamin C as ascorbic acid, 50-75 mg. should be started on the fifth day. A water-soluble vitamin D preparation in doses of 1000 to 2000 I.U. daily should be started about the seventh day.

7. Weight should be taken every second or third day as an indication of the baby's progress and as a criterion for increments in formula.
8. While oral feedings are being increased, infrequently one may have to administer parenteral fluids should the tissue turgor of the infant indicate presence of some dehydration. In view of the decreased clearance ability of the kidney for NaC1, the use of equal parts of 5% glucose in distilled water and lactate-Ringer's solution would be preferable to physiologic saline. If more than one clysis is administered, the above mixture might be alternated with 2½% glucose in distilled water. Amounts to be given, depending on the size of the baby and the apparent need for fluid, may vary from 15 to 40 c.c. by clysis one or more times a day. These procedures may be carried out in the incubator.
9. Vitamin K should be given all premature infants shortly after birth. Hykinone, 4.8 mg., or other vitamin K preparation may be used, and this may be repeated in 48 to 72 hours.

Care in Nursery—Cont'd

10. In a situation where a premature infant is not doing well even though no definite evidence of infection is detected, a diagnosis which may be difficult to make in a premature infant, one is justified in using penicillin and/or sulfa or preferably aureomycin or Chloromycetin. There are some reports concerning the use of penicillin or sulfa as a prophylactic measure in premature infants, though this is not generally recommended. For a premature infant not doing well, for which no adequate explanation can be determined, especially if respirations are irregular and infant at times apneic, the administration of blood may improve the general condition. Blood supplies the respiratory enzyme, carbonic anhydrase, in which premature infants are deficient, and also may help any anemia, hypoproteinemia, or tendency to edema.

The fundamental principles of care of the premature infant can be grouped under five general headings.

1. Maintenance of oxygenation.
2. Maintenance of optimal body temperature.
3. Prevention of infection.
4. Feeding for nutrition and growth.
5. Good nursing care.

The care of the premature infant must be individualized, each infant being a specific and particular problem. The smaller the infant, the greater the skill and more delicate handling required for successfully carrying out the fundamental principles of care of the premature infant as given above.

References

1. Levine, S. Z.: Introduction to the Problem of Prematurity, Am. J. Dis. Child. 73: 694, 1947.
2. Dunham, Ethel C.: Premature Infants, Childrens' Bureau Publication, 1948.
3. Gordon, Harry H.: Prematurity. Advances in Pediatrics, vol. II, New York, 1947, Interscience Publishers, Inc.

CHAPTER IX

MISCELLANEOUS EMERGENCIES

BITES

DOG BITE

The treatment of dog bites should conform with the regulations of the health department of each individual community. Nevertheless, the basic principles are included below.

1. Cleanse wound thoroughly with soap and water.
2. Cauterize* wound with fuming nitric acid (unless wound is on face).
3. Administer antirabies vaccine (Pasteur treatment) if
   (a) The dog is not available for observation.
   (b) The dog bite occurred on face or head.
   (c) The dog was rabid, even though the patient was only exposed but not bitten.
4. Tetanus toxoid or antitoxin should also be administered in usual doses.

HUMAN BITES

1. Cleanse wound thoroughly with soap and water.
2. Débride carefully.
3. Pack with zinc peroxide medicinal.
4. Chemotherapy and/or antibiotic therapy.

INSECT BITES

ANT BITES AND BEE STINGS[1]†

1. Prompt application of 5% ointment of Thephorin (Hoffmann-La Roche) with gentle massage alleviates pain and generally prevents local swelling.
2. The oral administration in usual therapeutic doses of one of the various antihistaminic agents may be of additional value.

---

*Surgical débridement with careful cleansing is considered by some to be equally efficacious and to be less injurious to local tissues.

†See also addendum, page 239.

BITES—Cont'd
INSECT BITES—Cont'd

BLACK WIDOW SPIDER BITE

The black widow spider, of the genus Latrodectus, is usually considered to be the only spider in the United States capable of causing serious symptoms.

The bite of only the female of the species causes the following symptoms:

1. In one to two hours, pain at the site of the bite.
2. Pain spreads to all the voluntary muscles of the body.
3. Abdominal cramps are severe and abdominal pain becomes excruciating.
4. Irritability.
5. Restlessness.
6. Headache.
7. Profuse perspiration.
8. Collapse.

Physical Findings

1. Boardlike rigidity of the abdomen.
2. Deep reflexes are hyperactive.
3. Only slight temperature elevation.
4. A small, red blotch may frequently be discovered. This represents the site of the bite.

Treatment

1. Hot tub baths afford some relief.
2. Morphine, 1/24 to 1/8 gr., depending on the size of the child.
3. 5-10 c.c. of 10% calcium gluconate, intravenously, may be given.
4. Specific therapy is *Latrodectus mactans* antivenin given intramuscularly. This affords relief from all symptoms within 1 to 2 hours. Dosage: 2.5 c.c. which may be repeated in 1-2 hours if symptoms are not relieved.

BITES—Cont'd
INSECT BITES—Cont'd
BLACK WIDOW SPIDER BITE—Cont'd
Treatment—Cont'd

5. The site of the bite should be cleansed to prevent secondary infection.
6. Tetanus antitoxin may be necessary. (See section on Tetanus, page 50.)

The untreated patient usually will recover in 24-48 hours, but several deaths have been reported.

TICK BITE

Tick bites are not infrequently encountered in pediatric practice in certain areas of the country. Generally, the tick is found embedded in the scalp or at the base of the head. Occasionally, one might encounter frank cases of tick paralysis which may require differentiation from either poliomyelitis or even botulism.

1. The tick should be removed as soon as possible with the use of a pair of forceps. 1 or 2 drops of kerosene, ether, or alcohol (at a point where the head is embedded in the skin) will facilitate removal.
2. The site of puncture must then be carefully cleansed and protected from possible secondary infection.

SNAKE BITE

A. Two main types of venoms.
   1. Neurotoxic—This form gives rise to pain at site of bite with slight edema. Dysphagia, myalgia, headaches, and drowsiness occur a few hours later.
   2. Hemorrhagic—This form gives rise to acute, burning pain associated with local swelling and discoloration.

B. Emergency snake bite kits available.
   1. In eastern U. S. A.
      (a) Snake Bite Outfit No. 2006, Becton, Dickinson and Co., Rutherford, N. J.

(b) Snake Bite First Aid Packet, David Equipment Co., New York, N. Y.

2. In southern U. S. A.
   (a) The Dudley Kit, Flack Hendrick Co., San Antonio, Texas.
3. In western U. S. A.
   (a) The Venex Snake Bite Kit, E. D. Bullard Co., San Francisco, Calif.
   (b) The Snake Bite First Aid Packet, Davis Emergency Equipment Co., San Francisco, Calif.

C. Apply ligature a short distance proximal to bite. (Pulse should be palpable with ligature in place.)

D. *Incision and suction.*—Although there is some difference in opinion about incising bite areas, it seems best to advise multiple incisions at site of fang marks. Suction should be applied for 20 minutes of each hour for several hours. (No potassium permanganate crystals should be applied to incision wounds.)
During intervals between suction, the incisions should be covered with sterile dressings previously saturated with either 2% sodium chloride or 2% magnesium sulfate. This hypertonic solution assists in local drainage.

E. *Antivenin therapy.*—This is undoubtedly the most important phase of snake bite therapy.
1. *Preparations available.* Lyovac Antivenin Nearctic Crotalidae (Sharpe & Dohme, Inc., Philadelphia, Pa.) This is a polyvalent serum against poison of rattlesnakes, copperheads, moccasins, and pit vipers.
2. *Precautions.* Usual eye and intradermal serum sensitivity tests should be done.
3. *Dose.* Because of greater concentration of venom per body weight, children require larger doses than adults. Inject ½ of the 15 c.c. vial at site of fang marks and the other half intramuscularly. Repeat at half-hour intervals until 60-70 c.c. have been given.

BITES—Cont'd
SNAKE BITES—Cont'd

F. *Supportive therapy.*

1. Avoid exercise to delay absorption of venom.
2. Transfusions to counteract hemorrhagic tendency.

BURNS

A. Home Treatment of Mild Burns

1. Local therapy. Petrolatum or any mild soothing ointment.
2. Analgesic. Aspirin in usual doses may be sufficient to obtund pain.

B. Hospital Treatment of Severe and Extensive Burns

In general, shock may be expected to develop in infants or children under 6 years of age who have 8% or more of the body surface affected and in children over 6 years of age who have 15% or more affected.

1. *General considerations.*
   (a) Maintain surgical cleanliness.
   (b) Employ antitetanus treatment as outlined in section on Tetanus (page 50).
   (c) Oxygen for dyspnea or cyanosis.
   (d) Hemoglobin and urine examination should be done.
   (e) Make a diagram of burned areas.[2] (See Figs. 9 and 10.)
   (f) It is necessary to treat for shock even before dressing the burns.
   (g) Record fluid intake and urine output daily.
2. *Analgesia.*
   (a) Morphine sulfate, 1/12 to 1/8 gr. on admission, or
   (b) Codeine sulfate, 1/4 to 1/2 gr. on admission.
3. *Systemic therapy.*
   (a) Shock therapy.[3]

BURNS—Cont'd

B. Hospital Treatment of Severe and Extensive Burns—Cont'd

3. *Systemic therapy*—Cont'd
   (a) Shock therapy—Cont'd

(1) Start initial dose of electrolyte* (30-40 drops per minute or faster if patient is in severe shock) and then follow with initial dose of plasma according to the plan given in Table IX.

TABLE IX.

WEIGHT (POUNDS)	10% DEXTROSE ELECTROLYTE IN SALINE SOLUTION (C.C.)	PLASMA (C.C.)
100-149	1000	500
50-99	500	250
35-49	250	250
20-34	150	150
5-19	20-50	10 per pound

(2) If shock persists or if blood pressure is down, repeat plasma.

(3) Do another hemoglobin determination. If hemoglobin has risen 10% or increased to 110% (i.e., if hemoconcentration is evident), give second dose of intravenous fluids and plasma as outlined in Table IX. (If this second administration of fluids is necessary during the first 24 hours, 10% dextrose in water should be used rather than 10% dextrose in saline.)

TABLE X. SUBSEQUENT AMOUNTS OF ELECTROLYTE AND PLASMA TO BE GIVEN FOR EACH POINT RISE IN HEMOGLOBIN OR FOR EACH POINT IT IS ABOVE 100 PER CENT ACCORDING TO THE WEIGHT OF THE PATIENT

WEIGHT (POUNDS)	10% DEXTROSE ELECTROLYTE IN DISTILLED WATER (C.C.)	PLASMA (C.C.)
100-149	35	35
50-99	20	20
35-49	15	15
20-34	10	10
5-19	0.5 per pound	0.5 per pound

*Use 10% dextrose electrolyte in saline solution. (To each 1000 c.c. of 10% dextrose in saline, add 3.75 Gm. of sodium bicarbonate, 1 Gm. of ascorbic acid, 2 ampules vitamin B complex.)

NAME ______________________________ AGE ____________

BURN RECORD AGES - BIRTH to 7½ YEARS DATE OF OBSERVATION ____________

RELATIVE PERCENTAGES OF AREAS AFFECTED BY GROWTH

AREA	AGE	0	1	5
A = 1/2 of Head		9½	8½	6½
B = 1/2 of One Thigh		2-3/4	3¼	4
C = 1/2 of One Leg		2½	2½	2-3/4

% BURN BY AREAS

Probable 3rd° Burn	Head ......Neck...... Body...... Up.Arm...... Forearm......Hands...... Genitals......Buttocks......Thighs........Legs......Feet ....
Total Burn	Head ......Neck...... Body......Up.Arm...... Forearm......Hands....... Genitals....... Buttocks........ Thighs ...... Legs.......Feet........

Sum of All Areas Probably 3rd° ____________ Total Burn ____________

Fig. 9.—Relative percentages of areas affected by growth—birth to 7½ years.

NAME ______________________ AGE __________

BURN RECORD AGES 7½ Yrs. to ADULT DATE OF OBSERVATION __________

RELATIVE PERCENTAGES OF AREAS AFFECTED BY GROWTH

AREA	AGE 10	15	Adult
A = 1/2 of Head	5½	4½	3½
B = 1/2 of One Thigh	4¼	4½	4-3/4
C = 1/2 of One Leg	3	3¼	3½

% BURN BY AREAS

Probable 3rd° Burn { Head...... Neck...... Body...... Up.Arm...... Forearm......Hands.......
Buttocks........Genitals...... Thighs.......Legs........ Feet.........

Total Burn { Head...... Neck...... Body...... Up.Arm...... Forearm......Hands.......
Genitals...... Buttocks...... Thighs...... Legs...... Feet ....

Sum of All Areas Probably 3rd° __________ Total Burn __________

Fig. 10.—Relative percentages of areas affected by growth—7½ years to adult.

BURNS—Cont'd

B. Hospital Treatment of Severe and Extensive Burns—Cont'd

3. *Systemic therapy*—Cont'd

(a) *Shock therapy*—Cont'd

(4) If more fluids are needed than outlined in Table X, use only plasma.

(5) Hemoglobin, temperature, and respirations should be done every 2 hours; blood pressure should be taken every half hour.

(6) Aqueous adrenal cortical extract should always be administered (see page 67).

(b) Barbiturates may be administered to control fear and nervousness.

(c) Prophlyactic penicillin, 400,000 units of fortified pencillin G in aqueous solution twice daily, given intramuscularly.

(d) Management of hyperpyrexia. Careful sponging or even ice water baths may be necessary to keep temperature below 102° F.

4. *Local therapy.* Pressure dressings should be used with sterile petrolatum except on face, neck, arms, and genitals, where simply sterile petrolatum is generally most useful.

ELECTRIC SHOCK

1. Free from current (use a nonconductor—wood, heavy rubber, plastic).
2. Artificial respiration. (Several hours may be needed to resuscitate the individual.)
3. Oxygen and oxygen CO_2 mixtures.
4. Caffeine with sodium benzoate is helpful as a respiratory stimulant. However, it must be given intravenously.
5. *Avoid epinephrine.*
6. After cardiorespiratory activity is restored, ephedrine sulfate may be of value to bolster blood pressure whenever the blood pressure is appreciably lowered.

EPISTAXIS

Treatment

Epistaxis may result from a variety of causes. Although the cause should be determined whenever epistaxis occurs frequently, the following methods may be used to control acute bleeding.

1. Local pressure.
   (a) Simple nasal compression.
   (b) Packing of the anterior nares with a rubber finger cot stuffed with gauze (a short string should be attached to the finger cot so that it may be easily withdrawn).
   (c) Packing of the posterior nares with absorbable, oxidized cellulose.
2. Local ice application.
   (a) Place over the nose.
   (b) Small piece of ice may be introduced into the nostrils.
   (c) Reflex capillary contraction may be brought about by
      (1) Application of ice to the back of the neck or
      (2) placing ice chips in the mouth.
3. Local medicaments.
   (a) Powdered rabbit thrombin, human fibrinogen, oxidized, cellulose, or gelatin foam.
   (b) Adrenalin, ephedrine, or hydrogen peroxide may be useful.
   (c) Cauterize with chromic acid on a metal applicator with moistened cotton so that no undissolved crystals adhere to the nostril. Do not cauterize both sides of the septum simultaneously.
4. Supportive measures.
   (a) Administration of vitamin K parenterally, 4.8 mg.
   (b) Whole blood or fresh plasma.

EPISTAXIS—Cont'd
Treatment—Cont'd
4. Supportive measures—Cont'd

(c) Fresh platelet transfusion, if available.
(d) Antibiotics to control infection.

EYE INJURIES, ACCIDENTS, AND FOREIGN BODIES

A. FOREIGN BODIES (Nonpenetrating)

1. Rub the unaffected eye gently to produce lacrimation of both eyes.
2. Irrigate affected eye with clean water, normal saline, or 1% boric acid solution.
3. If above procedures have not cleared eye of foreign substance, attempt to remove body by lightly passing a moistened cotton pledget over conjunctival sac.
4. If foreign body is still present, use
   (a) Local anesthetic (Butyn 1%).
   (b) Fine horsehair loop to remove body.

B. FOREIGN BODIES (Penetrating)

1. Apply eye pad and head bandage.
2. Request immediate care by ophthalmologist.

C. CHEMICAL BURNS

1. General considerations.
   (a) Testing. If nature of foreign chemical is not definitely known, test contents of conjunctival sac with either alkacid test paper or pHydrion paper.* (Litmus paper is not reliable because a large pH shift is required before a color change from the blue to red or from red to blue occurs.)
   (b) Irrigate eye with copious amounts of water or saline.

---

*Available through Physician's Drug and Supply Company, 3rd and Callowhill Streets, Philadelphia 6, Pa., and Micro Essential Labs., Brooklyn, N. Y.

EYE INJURIES, ACCIDENTS, AND FOREIGN BODIES—Cont'd
C. CHEMICAL BURNS—Cont'd
1. General considerations—Cont'd

(c) Instill local anesthetic: 1% Butyn, 1% Pontocaine, or 1% Holocaine.
(d) Continue irrigation with water or isotonic saline for at least one-half hour unless specific neutralizing solutions, as listed below, are available.
(e) If insoluble particles are present, remove promptly by swabbing from the conjunctival sac or the corneal epithelium.

ALTHOUGH NEUTRALIZING SOLUTIONS ARE LISTED BELOW, EQUALLY GOOD RESULTS HAVE BEEN OBTAINED IN ALL CHEMICAL BURNS OF EYES FOLLOWING IMMEDIATE IRRIGATION WITH COPIOUS AMOUNTS OF TAP WATER

2. *Acid burns.*
(a) 3 to 4 c.c. of a 2% solution of sodium bicarbonate should be instilled over eyeball and into conjunctival sac every 3 to 5 minutes. This is continued until contents of conjunctival sacs at fornices give neutral reaction.
(b) Instill local anesthetic together with oily lubricant and some bacteriostatic substance liberally.

Products most useful.
(1) Butyn and Metaphen ointment (this is a rapid but short-acting anesthetic).
(2) Metycaine and Merthiolate ointment (this is a slower but more prolonged acting anesthetic).
(3) Boric acid and ophthalmic ointment.
(4) Sterile castor oil, cod liver oil, or olive oil.

(c) Dark glasses, eye pads, and atropine (or homatropine) should be used as suggested by an ophthalmologist who should see all these cases in consultation.

EYE INJURIES, ACCIDENTS, AND FOREIGN BODIES—Cont'd
C. Chemical Burns—Cont'd

3. *Alkali burns.*
   (a) 3-5 c.c. of a 1% acetic acid solution should be instilled over eyeball and into conjunctival sacs every 3-5 minutes for 30-50 minutes, or longer, until contents of conjunctival sacs at fornices give neutral reaction.
   (b) Apply cold compresses.
   (c) Instill local anesthetic together with oily lubricant and some bacteriostatic substance liberally. For products most useful, see (b) under Acid Burns.
   (d) Dark glasses, eye pads, and atropine (or homatropine) should be used as recommended by an ophthalmologist who should see all these cases in consultation.
4. Alkaloid burns.
   (a) 3-5 of a 3% solution of sodium thiosulfate should be instilled over the eyeball and into the conjunctival sac every 3-5 minutes for 30-50 minutes.
   (b) Further therapy as outlined above under Alkali Burns.
5. *Lime burns.*
   (a) Irrigate eye with a freshly prepared 5 or 10% solution of neutral ammonium tartrate.

FROSTBITE

Signs and Symptoms

1. First degree (mild).
   (a) Outer layers of skin involved with no blistering or peeling.
   (b) Waxy pallor usual. May also be yellow or purple discoloration.
   (c) Numbness or paresthesia.
   (d) Symptoms subside on warming or upon return to normal environment.

FROSTBITE—Cont'd
Signs and Symptoms—Cont'd
1. First degree (mild)—Cont'd

(e) Hypersensitivity to further exposure to cold for months thereafter.

2. Second degree (moderate).
   (a) Death to superficial layers of skin.
   (b) Tissues firm; digits stiff.
   (c) Blistering or peeling.
   (d) Edema.
   (e) Superficial layers appear necrotic.
   (f) Pain of burning character.
   (g) Reactive hyperemia on thawing.
   (h) Heal with scarring.
3. Third degree (marked).
   (a) Death to deep layers of skin, subcutaneous tissue, and upper muscular layers.
   (b) Desquamation at ends of involved digits.
   (c) Loss of sensation. No pain.
   (d) Prostration with high fever.
4. Fourth degree (severe).
   (a) Death to deep muscles and bone.
   (b) Gangrene resulting in loss of extremity or portion thereof.
   (c) Systemic reaction with high fever and prostration.

Treatment

Mild

1. Loosen all tightly fitting garments.
2. Return to warm environment.
3. Do not apply additional heat.

More Severe Types

These are emergencies and therapy must be instituted early to prevent or minimize thrombosis.

FROSTBITE—Cont'd
Treatment—Cont'd

Immediate Treatment

1. Warm by body contact heat.
2. Do NOT use affected part.
3. Do NOT rub or traumatize skin.
4. Do NOT apply snow.
5. Apply sterile dressings over area involved.
6. Hospitalize.

Hospital Treatment

1. Warm extremity slowly without exposure to heat greater than natural room temperature.
2. Paint extremity with mild antiseptic (Merthiolate 1:5000, Acriflavine 1:1000). Cover with sterile dressing.
3. Raise affected part on pillow, or elevate by suspension.
4. Tetanus antitoxin 1,500 units (after proper testing as outlined in section on Tetanus, page 50), or Tetanus toxoid plain, 1 c.c., if child has had active immunization.
5. Antibiotics systemically.
   (a) Penicillin, 25,000 to 50,000 units in aqueous solution every three hours, or 200,000 to 400,000 units of "fortified" procaine penicillin intramuscularly once daily.
   (b) Sulfonamide, 1 gr. per pound per day.
6. Anticoagulants. These keep interstitial fluid with all its constituents resorbable.
   (a) Heparin (intravenously).
      (1) Initial dose, 0.5 mg. per kilogram.
      (2) It requires about the same amount of heparin per hour to keep the clotting time at a given length as it does to prolong it to that extent.
      Example: A child weighing 10 kilograms would get 5 mg. heparin stat, and this would be followed by approximately 5 mg. during each hour.

FROSTBITE—Cont'd
Treatment—Cont'd
Hospital Treatment—Cont'd
6. Anticoagulants—Cont'd
(a) Heparin (intravenously)—Cont'd

(3) Keep clotting time between 20-30 minutes until the danger of thrombosis has passed (6 days)—best accomplished by adding heparin to a continuous intravenous drip of normal saline or 5% glucose. By adjusting the rate of flow, the amount of heparin can be regulated and the clotting time can be maintained between 20-30 minutes.
(4) Periodic determinations of clotting time imperative.
(5) In cases of bleeding, give small blood transfusions.
(b) Dicumarol.
(1) Delayed action of 48 hours disadvantageous.
7. Warm drinks. Alcohol: 1 dram to ½ ounce of whiskey in sugar water.
8. Sedation.
(a) Phenobarbital or pentobarbital, ¼ to ½ gr. every 4 hours as needed.
(b) Antihistaminics of Benadryl type for smooth muscle relaxation, sedation, and cold sensitivity (hives) if it occurs. Dose, 2 to 4 mg. per pound per day. (Antihistaminics of tripelennamine type act as spasmogenic agent.)
9. Other measures.
(a) Sympathetic block or paravertebral block with 1% procaine.
(b) Peripheral vasodilators.
Adrenolytic and sympatholytic vasodilators.
(1) Tetra-ethyl ammonium chloride, "TEA" (Etamon—Parke-Davis). Improves cutaneous sensation, and relieves symptoms due to circulatory insufficiency.

FROSTBITE—Cont'd
Treatment—Cont'd
Hospital Treatment—Cont'd
9. Other measures—Cont'd
(b) Peripheral vasodilators—Cont'd
Adrenolytic and sympatholytic vasodilators—Cont'd
(1) Tetra-ethyl ammonium chloride, "TEA"—Cont'd

Dose: *Intravenous,* not to exceed 7 mg. per kilogram.
Intramuscular, 5 to 10 (not to exceed 20) mg. per kilogram.

(2) Benzylimidazoline hydrochloride (Priscoline—Ciba)
Dose: Orally or intramuscularly
Adolescents, 50 mg.
Children over 5 years, 25 mg.
Children under 5 years, 10 mg.
Increase by 10 mg. every 4 hours until flushing or "goose flesh" appear.

(c) Wet penicillin dressings, 500 to 1000 units per cubic centimeter.
(d) Pressure dressings and casts.
(e) Therapeutic refrigerator, 2 to 3° C. for 1 week.

10. Surgical consultation.
Restrain hasty amputation because of blackened skin. All attempts should be made to minimize loss of extremity, and every chance should be given the extremity to return to normal, even if it takes months.

HEAT EXHAUSTION

Symptoms

Weakness, dizziness, stupor, pallor, perspiration, tachycardia, tachypnea, hypotension, hypothermia, or moderate elevation (101° F.).

HEAT EXHAUSTION—Cont'd

Treatment

1. Rest in cool place.
2. Cool sponges or warm baths to return temperature to normal.
3. Glucose and saline should be given orally or parenterally.

Note: It has been demonstrated that heat prostration may be prevented by the administration of 100 mg. of ascorbic acid orally daily.

HEATSTROKE AND SUNSTROKE

Symptoms

Headache, dizziness, nausea, unconsciousness, skin flushed, dry or hot. Marked hyperthermia (108-109° F.).

Treatment

1. Spray body with cool water and massage limbs briskly.
2. Increase evaporation by fanning or by use of electric fan.
3. Constant care to avoid development and early treatment of pulmonary congestion which may supervene.

HEMORRHAGE

Acute hemorrhage demanding emergency treatment may result from a variety of causes.

1. Traumatic.
2. Postoperative.
3. Spontaneous (due to an undiagnosed cause).
4. Blood dyscrasias.

The bleeding may be superficial or hidden. Shock may be present or supervene shortly.

The emergency treatment is essentially the same:

HEMORRHAGE--Cont'd

1. Attempt to stop the bleeding.
   - (a) Local pressure.
   - (b) Hemostatic agents.
     - (1) Powdered rabbit thrombin.
     - (2) Human fibrinogen.
     - (3) Oxidized cellulose.
     - (4) Gelatine foam.
2. Type and cross-match patient's blood.
3. Administer plasma or whole blood. If neither is immediately available, administer 5% glucose in saline while obtaining plasma and/or whole blood.
4. Specific agents for bleeding due to blood dyscrasias.
   - (a) Thrombocytopenic purpura.
     - (1) Fresh platelet transfusions, if available, are frequently useful in acute episodes.
   - (b) Hemophilia.
     - (1) Fresh whole blood or fresh plasma transfusions are of real value in hemophilia.
     - (2) It may be stated that during active bleeding fresh blood or plasma should be given every 12 hours because the reduction in coagulation time following plasma infusion lasts for about 12 to 14 hours.
     - (3) It should be emphasized that local application of hemostatic agents, such as those listed above, is only of value if applied directly to the bleeding points rather than merely to the wound.
     - (4) Antihemophilic globulin may be used if available. Its administration, including dosage, should depend on the preparation available.
     - (5) Rest and quiet.
     - (6) Acute hemarthrosis in hemophilia:
       - (i) Treat as above.
       - (ii) The joints should be in a position of maximum relaxation.

(iii) The local application of ice packs may afford relief of discomfort and reduce bleeding.
(iv) Analgesics and opiates may be necessary to control marked discomfort.
(v) Apply compression bandages before too much swelling occurs.

HICCOUGH

Hiccough is a common occurrence in infancy. Generally, it is not of sufficient severity to require medical aid. Furthermore, most of the episodes are self-limited. Nevertheless, severe, persistent episodes may occasionally be encountered in older children. These frequently require some type of medical treatment. Because of the multitude of causative factors, there are many different methods of treatment. Not infrequently several methods must be used before the attack is terminated. Some of the treatments, listed subsequently, require the cooperation of the patient; thus, these will not be applicable in a young child who cannot cooperate sufficiently by following suggestions.

Treatment

1. Hold the breath (forced expiration will be of value).
2. Drink cold liquid slowly, with continuous, prolonged swallowing.
3. Pressure on the phrenic nerve between the two heads of the sternocleidomastoid muscle.
4. Stimulate cough reflex by tickling the soft palate.
5. Pressure on the eyeballs.
6. Gastric lavage (this includes deflation of dilated stomach which may be the cause of hiccough in the postoperative period).

HICCOUGH—Cont'd
Treatment—Cont'd

7. Inhalation of amyl nitrite from a small perle.
8. Cautious inhalation of ammonia vapor.
9. Inhalation of carbon dioxide for several minutes
   (a) From common supply cylinder.
   (b) From bag containing a piece of dry ice in 1 to 2 ounces of water.
10. The use of quinidine sulfate has recently been recommended in the severe, protracted cases of hiccough which do not respond to other measures. The dosage recommended in the therapy of paroxysmal tachycardia (page 20) may be used.

PEDIATRIC ANESTHESIA

This subject has developed into a science of its own. Certain excellent reference sources are now available.[4, 5] The basic principles of respiratory physiology and resuscitation should be carefully understood. Emphasis will be placed in this section on the preanesthetic medication phase of pediatric anesthesia.

Although there is no general agreement on dosage schedules of analgesics, sedatives, and hypnotics in pediatrics, certain well-established features of anesthesia in children may be listed.

1. The margin of safety in infants and children is considerably less than in adults.
2. Strict attention to detail is more important than in adults.
3. It is most important to put the infant or child at ease as much as possible.
   (a) Intelligent psychotherapy makes for good induction for good anesthesia.
4. Proper appraisal of the physical condition of the patient is essential.
   (a) Deficiencies in hydration and electrolyte balance should be corrected.

(b) Make sure that no marked anemia exists.
(c) Always check urine for acetone and sugar to eliminate diabetes.

5. Preanesthetic medication.
   (a) Common agents used.
      (1) Opiates: Codeine, morphine, Demerol
      (2) Barbiturates: Phenobarbital, pentobarbital, Seconal, Amytal.
      (3) Belladonna derivatives and related compounds: Atropine, scopolamine.
   (b) The dosages used are based on certain individual factors.
      (1) The apparent age of the child.
      (2) Type of anesthetic agent chosen and type of anesthesia.
      (3) General condition of patient including state of hydration and presence of acidosis.

      The dosages in Table XI[5] may be used.
   (c) Time of administration.
      (1) Barbiturates and opiates should be given, whenever possible, 1 to 1½ hours prior to induction of anesthesia.
      (2) Belladonna derivatives should be given ½ hour before anesthesia.
   (d) Special considerations.
      (1) Respiratory depression may be caused by opiates in the very sick child or in the newborn infant.
      (2) Combinations of 2 of the agents listed in Table XI are frequently made. It is well to point out, however, that frequently combinations which include morphine are less desirable than those not including morphine.

TABLE XI. DOSAGE OF DRUGS FOR PREANESTHETIC MEDICATION*

(From Nelson, editor: Mitchell-Nelson Textbook of Pediatrics, 1950.[5])

AGE	WEIGHT		MORPHINE (SUBCUT.)		DEMEROL (SUBCUT.)		ATROPINE† (SUBCUT.)		SECONAL‡ (RECTALLY)	
	POUNDS	KG.	GR.	MG.	GR.	MG.	GR.	MG.	GR.	MG.
Birth	7.4	3.3	1/500	0.12	1/15	4	1/2500	0.025	1/3	20
3 mo.	12.7	5.7	1/300	0.2	1/9	7	1/1500	0.04	1/2	30
To 6 mo.	17	7.7	1/200	0.3	1/7	9	1/1000	0.06	3/4	45
To 12 mo.	22.4	10.2	1/120	0.5	1/5	12	1/600	0.1	1	60
To 2 yr.	27.7	13.0	1/100	0.6	1/4	15	1/500	0.12	1-1/2	90
To 3 yr.	33.7	15.3	1/60	1.0	1/3	20	1/400	0.15	2	120
To 5 yr.	40.9	18.6	1/50	1.2	2/5	25	1/350	0.18	3	150
To 8 yr.	55.5	25.2	1/32	1.8	3/5	37	1/300	0.20	2-1/2	180
To 12 yr.	80.9	36.7	1/20	3	4/5	50	1/150	0.4	2-3/4	200
To 14 yr.	100.3	45.5	1/12	5	1-1/4	75	1/150	0.4	3	200

*The extremely small dosages of preanesthetic drugs for infants require properly diluted solutions for accurate dosage.
†The dosage of Scopolamine can be calculated by taking two-thirds of the atropine dosage.
‡Dosage for sodium pentobarbital (Nembutal) and Sodium Amytal are the same as those given for Seconal.

PEDIATRIC ANESTHESIA—Cont'd

5. Preanesthetic medication—Cont'd

(d) Special considerations—Cont'd

(3) It must be remembered that Demerol has atropine-like actions, so that when it is combined with atropine the latter should be used in approximately ½ the quantity listed in Table XI.

6. The postoperative care of patients is as important as is the preanesthetic phase.
   (a) Ensure a continued good airway.
   (b) Place the patient in a warmed bed in a lateral position in slight Trendelenberg.
   (c) The patient's head should be kept extended and the lower jaw kept forward with mouth slightly open.
   (d) If hoarseness develops or if there is some difficulty in respirations, provide oxygen and high humidity. Suction the trachea frequently. Tracheotomy may occasionally be necessary.

SERUM REACTIONS*

A. Epinephrine, 2-3 minims of a 1:1000 solution subcutaneously.

B. Antihistaminics (Benadryl or Pyribenzamine, 2-3 mg. per pound) either prophylactically or as soon as first signs appear.

C. Procaine.

Indications

1. If serum or transfusion reactions persist over prolonged period.
2. If other methods listed above have not proved effective.
3. If persistent pyrexia is due to the reaction and not to infection.

Contraindications

1. If epinephrine or barbiturates previously used have not been fully metabolized or excreted.

---

*See also addendum, page 239.

SERUM REACTIONS—Cont'd
C. Procaine—Cont'd

Methods and Dosage

1. An 0.1% solution in normal saline of procaine hydrochloride is prepared under sterile precautions.
2. Total quantity to be given is calculated on the basis of 4 c.c. per kilogram of body weight.
3. The calculated amount is given intravenously in a 20-minute period.

Treatment of Toxicity

1. Stop procaine infusion (usually sufficient to control early toxic manifestations).
2. Sodium Amytal intravenously.
3. Oxygen.
4. Artificial respiration if necessary.

TRANSFUSION REACTIONS

Any one of five types may occur. They may be immediate or delayed.

A. *Immediate Reactions*

1. *Allergic.*
   (a) Cause. Sensitivity of recipient to some allergen in donor's blood.
   (b) Symptoms.
      (1) Urticaria.
      (2) Angioneurotic edema.
      (3) Asthma.
      (4) Anaphylactic shock.
   (c) Treatment.
      (1) *Prophylactic.* Antihistamine substances such as Benadryl or Pyribenzamine, 2-3 mg. per pound in divided doses for 24 hours prior to transfusion.

TRANSFUSION REACTIONS—Cont'd
A. *Immediate Reactions*—Cont'd
1. *Allergic*—Cont'd
(c) Treatment—Cont'd

(2) *Active.* Epinephrine (1:1000), 2-3 minims. Benadryl, 2 to 3 mg. per pound, or Pyribenzamine 2-3 mg. per pound.

2. *Pyrogenic.*
(a) Cause.
Contaminant—A bacterial product.
(b) Symptoms
(1) Mild fever and chills.
(2) Thermal center upset.
(c) Treatment.
(1) *Prophylactic.* Use of pyrogen-free equipment.
(2) *Active.* Antipyretic measures:
(i) Aspirin.
(ii) Cold packs.

3. *Hemolytic.*
(a) Cause. Any variety of blood incompatibility.
(b) *Clinical Course*[6]

I. "Reaction Shock" (First Day)	II. Renal Insufficiency (First-Twelfth Day)	III. Salt-Losing Diuresis (Eighth-Sixteenth Day)
Hemolysis and Hypotension	Tubular damage	Tubular recovery or regeneration
1. Sudden onset	1. Oliguria, heme casts	1. Copious diuresis
2. Apprehension, backache, etc.	2. Azotemia and hypertension	2. Severe dehydration if water and salt not supplied
3. Dyspnea, cyanosis	3. Elevated serum K	3. Recovery
4. Hypotension, mental confusion	4. Depressed serum Na, Cl, CO_2, CP, Ca	
5. Chill, fever	5. Rising titers of agglutinins and cryptagglutinoids	
6. Hemoglobinemia, hemoglobinuria		

TRANSFUSION REACTIONS—Cont'd
A. *Immediate Reactions*—Cont'd
3. *Hemolytic*—Cont'd

(c) *Therapy*[6]

(First Day)	(First-Twelfth Day)	(Eighth-Sixteenth Day)
1. Anemia, decreased blood volume and hypotension are treated with adequate amounts of compatible whole blood and plasma	1. Limit fluid (by mouth) intake to amount equal to estimated insensible water loss and urine output. Thus no attempt is made to force damaged kidneys into action 2. Use water-soluble vitamins C and B parenterally 3. CO_2 of plasma, Na, K, and Cl should be checked and deficits treated accordingly.	1. Replace water and salts lost in the urine as near as possible on a gram for gram basis by measuring urine volume and salt output

B. *Delayed Reactions*
1. Allergic—same as in Immediate Reactions.
2. Homologous serum jaundice or hepatitis.
This reaction is mentioned here only to emphasize that transfusions of plasma or whole blood are occasionally not without dire consequences unless special care has been maintained during the preparation of these agents. Thus, they should be given only when absolutely necessary.

SHOCK*

Shock may develop during any one of the emergency situations previously presented in this book. The various causative factors are presented in Table XII, adapted from the work of Moon.[6]

It is well to emphasize that, even more true in infants than in adults, there is great difficulty in recognizing the incipient stage of shock. Whenever the problem arises, it must be remembered that simple examinations such as RBC counts, hemoglobin determination, or hematocrit determination may be of real value in demonstrating hemoconcentration or hemo-

*See also addendum, page 241, and Table XIII, page 240.

TABLE XII. SUMMARY OF THE PATHOGENESIS OF SHOCK

(Adapted from Moon: Shock: Its Dynamics, Occurrence and Management, 1942.[6])

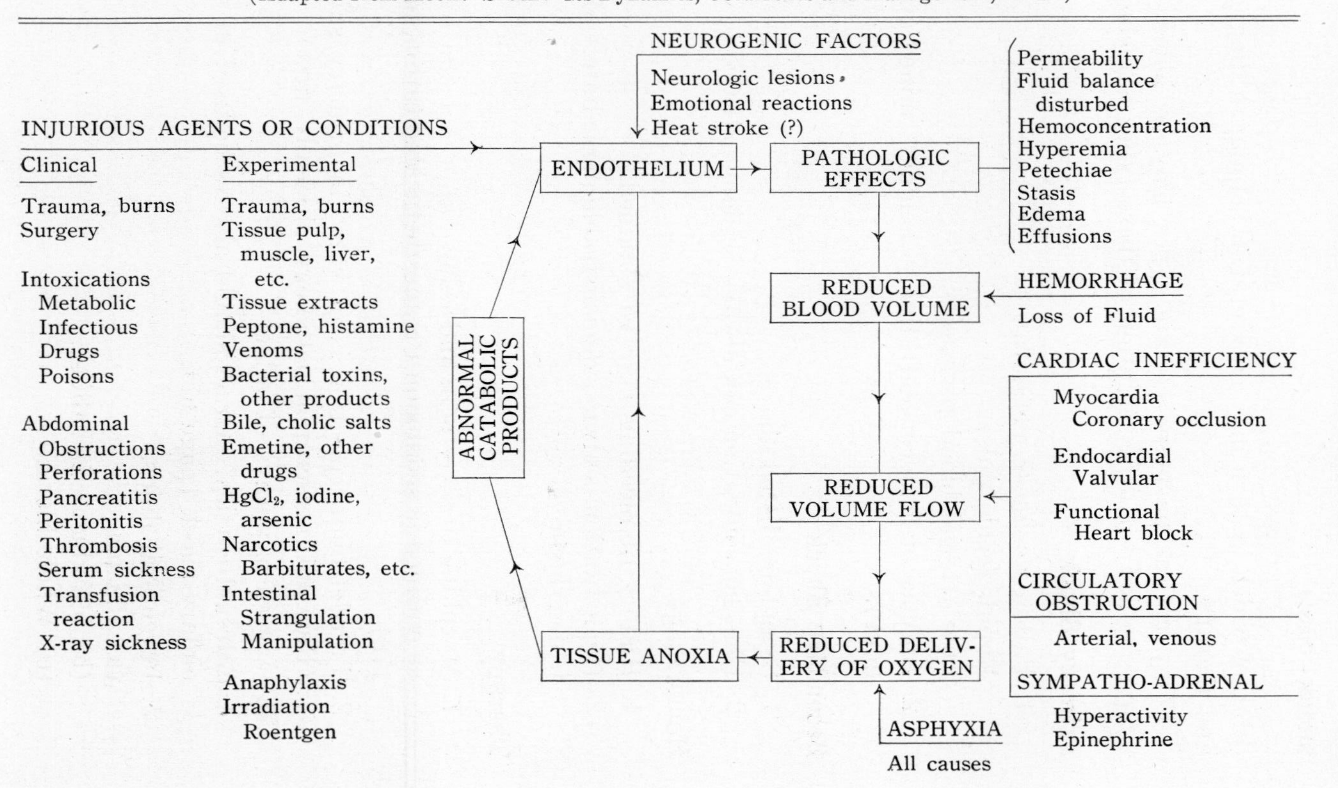

SHOCK—Cont'd

dilution which in turn may be useful in helping in diagnosis and therapy.

For practical purposes certain types may be listed. A simple method for differentiation of these types is included.

Primary Shock

1. Pallor, weakness, perspiration.
   Rapid, feeble pulse.
   Low arterial blood pressure.
2. Absence of hemoconcentration (when determined every hour).

Secondary Shock

1. Symptoms listed above.
2. Hemoconcentration can always be demonstrated.

Hemorrhage

1. History of bleeding may be obtained.
2. Hemodilution is always demonstrable immediately after hemorrhage.

Therapy

1. Morphine to allay pain and relieve apprehension (dose as outlined in section on Preanesthetic Medication, page 176).
2. Trendelenburg position is of value in primary shock. (Rule out intracranial pathology, clinically, first).
3. Oxygen is always of value.
4. Adrenal cortical extract should always be used in secondary shock (page 67).
5. Parenteral fluids.
   (a) Plasma.
   (b) 5% glucose in saline.
   (c) Whole blood.

References

1. Strauss, W. T.: Antihistamine Therapy of Bee Stings, J.A.M.A. **140**: 603, 1949.
2. Lund, C. C., and Browder, N. C.: The Estimation of Area of Burns, Surg., Gynec. and Obst. **79**: 352, 1944.
3. Levenson, S. M., et al.: An Outline for the Treatment of Severe Burns, New England J. Med. **235**: 76, 1946.
4. Leigh, M.D., and Belton, M. D.: Pediatric Anesthesia, New York, 1948, The Macmillan Co.
5. Nelson, W. E. (editor): Mitchell-Nelson Textbook of Pediatrics, ed. 5, Philadelphia, 1950, W. B. Saunders Co.
6. Moon, V. H.: Shock: Its Dynamics, Occurrence and Management, Philadelphia, 1942, Lea & Febiger.

CHAPTER X

PEDIATRIC PROCEDURES

Introduction

A knowledge of the technique of various procedures is often essential in the management of emergency conditions.

Although special problems will be discussed subsequently, certain common points may be emphasized.

1. Proper restraint of the patient is essential in all cases before any procedure is attempted. Although a variety of methods may be and are used for restraining infants and children, the methods generally employed by us are presented in Figs. 11, 12, and 13. The sheet is wrapped around the patient in such a manner that both extremities are at the sides and firmly restrained. These restraints are generally used when procedures are to be done wherein the neck or scalp structures are to be used.
2. Gentle handling of all patients is, of course, always indicated.

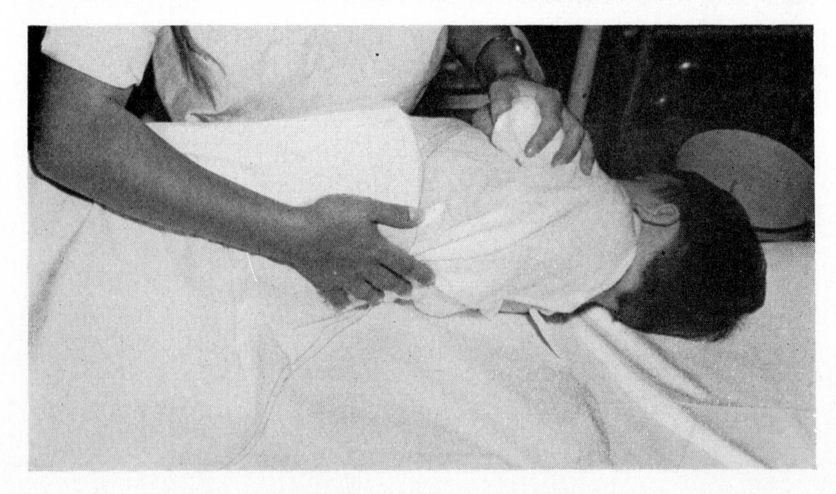

Fig. 11.—Proper restraint of patients—Step 1.

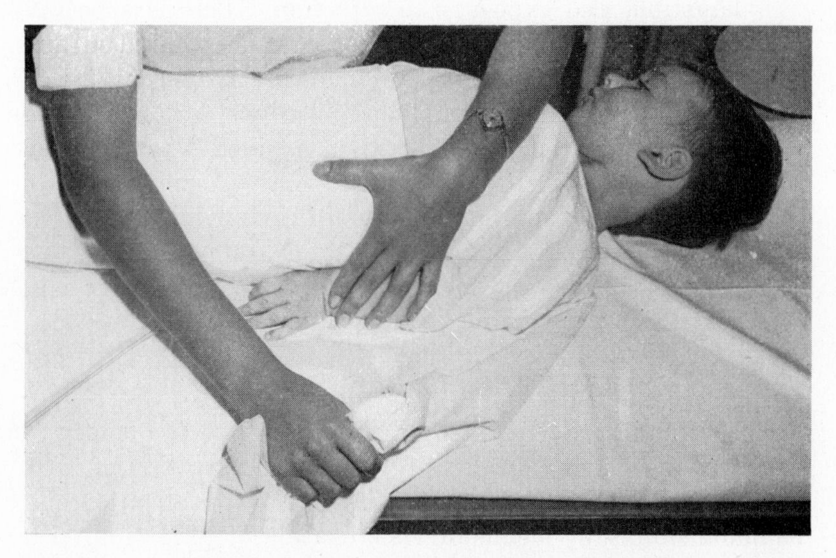

Fig. 12.—Proper restraint of patients—Step 2.

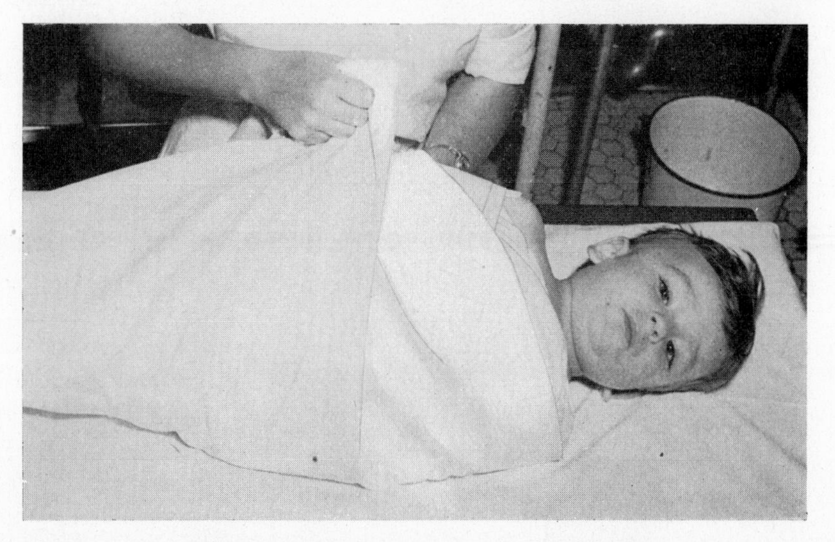

Fig. 13.—Proper restraint of patients—Step 3.

3. Special attention must be directed to avoid chilling, exhaustion, and exposure to infection. This is especially true in all newborn, premature, and debilitated infants.
4. Strict care for aseptic technique is always essential.
5. Potential hazards and complications of procedures should be anticipated and thus avoided whenever possible. It should be emphasized that whenever possible or necessary the operator should review important anatomic landmarks and relationships for each procedure. The difficulties one may encounter as well as the complications must be clearly recognized.

CUBITAL VEIN PUNCTURE

The veins in the cubital fossa are used quite frequently for withdrawing blood as well as for the administration of intravenous fluids and medications. Anatomic localization may be made simply by means of visualization or palpation. Fig. 14 presents the most common position of the available vessels and their relationships.

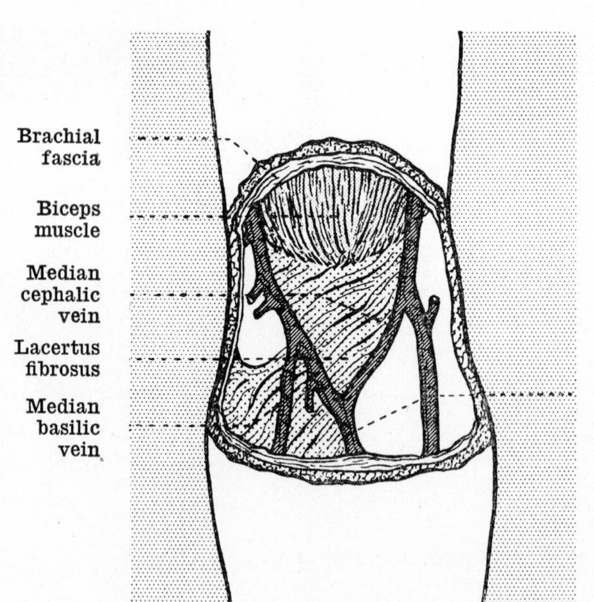

Fig. 14.—Anatomy of the antecubital space.

CUBITAL VEIN PUNCTURE—Cont'd

Although this method is most generally adaptable for older children, reasonable success may be achieved even in infants.

1. The arm should be restrained properly. One method is shown in Fig. 23.
   (a) An armboard is quite useful. It may be prepared easily by padding two strips of wood with gauze and adhesive tape. The arm board should be fastened to the bed with gauze strips, towel clips, or safety pins. The latter method has been used in the illustration but the pins are not visible.
   (b) Another method for immobilizing the arm and forearm is the use of sandbags to which the extremity is taped. This method is generally preferred if the physician does not have sufficient nursing assistance during the procedure.
2. A tourniquet should be placed as close as possible proximal to the site of the puncture.
3. A sharp, short-bevel needle is generally essential and always helpful. The needle should be closely examined for burrs; if present, the needle should not be used. No. 25 gauge to No. 20 needles may be used. The apparent size of the vessel and the nature of the procedure should be considered in the determination of the size of needle to be used. Naturally, a large needle is not preferred for a small vein. However, the smaller caliber needles are not generally preferred when blood is to be withdrawn for diagnostic purposes in large quantities or when a fluid of relatively high viscosity (such as blood) is to be administered intravenously by the constant drip method.
4. Tension on the skin distal to the point of puncture is helpful.
5. Mild, negative pressure in the syringe is important as soon as the skin has been punctured.

6. If a venipuncture is performed in order to obtain a blood specimen, the tourniquet should always be removed before the needle is withdrawn from the vein; pressure should be applied at the site of puncture for several minutes to avoid subcutaneous hematoma formation.
7. If the venipuncture is for therapeutic purposes, the needle should be made secure in the vein. Extravasation should be avoided. Thrombophlebitis should be anticipated whenever prolonged intravenous therapy is maintained at the same site. Thus, alternate vessels should be used as frequently as possible.

EXTERNAL JUGULAR VEIN PUNCTURE

Venipuncture of this vessel is most commonly performed for diagnostic purposes in infants. Rarely, in cases of shock, this vessel may serve temporarily as a site for intravenous fluid administration such as glucose, saline, and plasma.

The anatomic position and the proper position for the procedure is demonstrated in Figs. 15, 16, and 17.

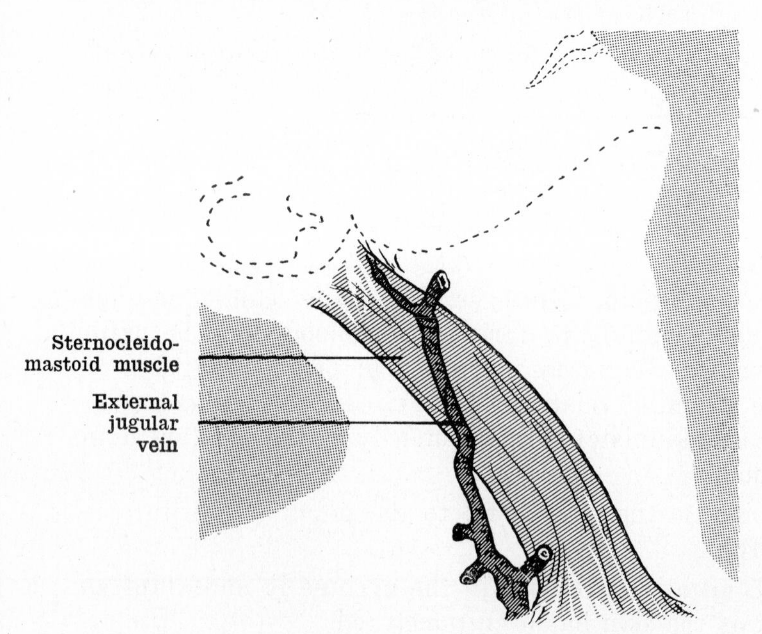

Fig. 15.—Superficial anatomy and course of the external jugular vein.

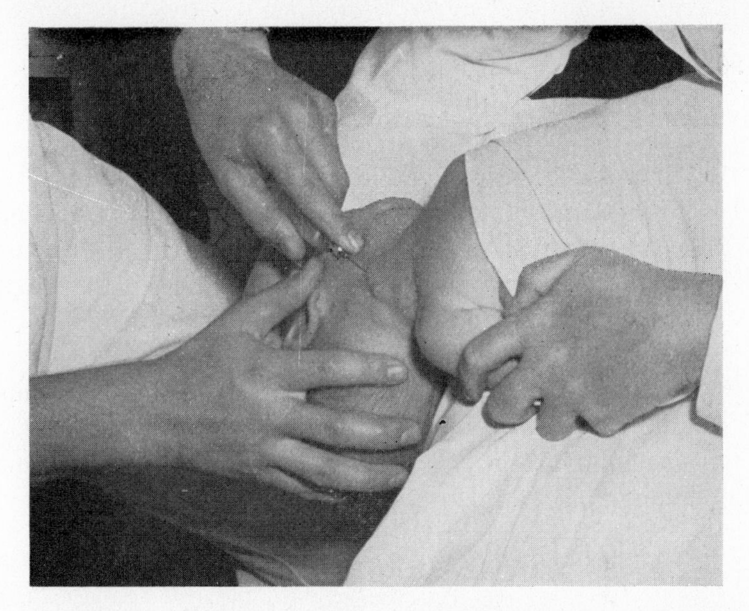

Fig. 16.—External jugular vein puncture (using finger as guide to palpate landmarks).

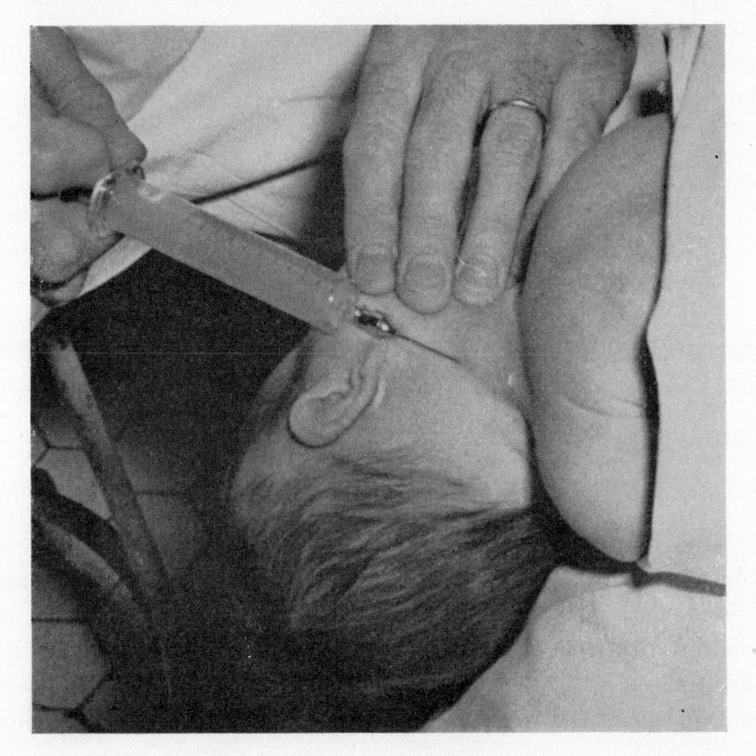

Fig. 17.—External jugular vein puncture (negative pressure of plunger in barrel is maintained on entering skin).

EXTERNAL JUGULAR VEIN PUNCTURE—Cont'd

1. Firm restraint is mandatory. The head should be held lower than the body with the head turned to the side.
2. A sharp, short-bevel needle is useful. Generally No. 20 or No. 22 gauge needles are applicable. The suggestions listed under Cubital Vein Puncture above (point 3) should be followed.
3. Hematoma formation at the puncture site is common unless local pressure is applied for several minutes.
4. The inadvertent introduction of air is to be cautiously avoided.

FEMORAL VEIN PUNCTURE

Puncture of the femoral vein is generally performed for diagnostic purposes. It may be performed with the patient in a position shown in Fig. 18. Nevertheless, one must briefly review the anatomy of this area before attempting femoral vein puncture. The femoral vein lies medial to the femoral artery below the inguinal ligament, as is shown in Fig. 19.

1. Palpate the femoral artery.
2. Insert a No. 20 or No. 22 gauge needle directly medial to the femoral artery approximately one inch below the inguinal ligament.
3. The needle should not be directed too cephalad in order to avoid puncture of any abdominal structures.
4. Firm, continuous pressure is essential after withdrawal of the needle to avoid hematoma formation.

INTERNAL JUGULAR VEIN PUNCTURE

This vessel is used much less frequently now than heretofore, especially since femoral vein technique has been more widely accepted as a routine procedure. Nevertheless, under certain circustances it may be necessary to use this vessel for withdrawing blood for diagnostic purposes. *This method is not intended for the administration of fluids or medications.*

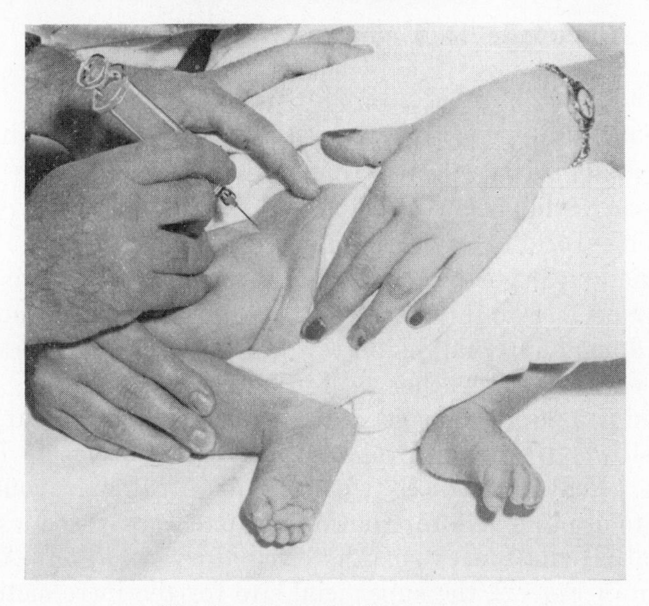

Fig. 18.—Femoral vein puncture.

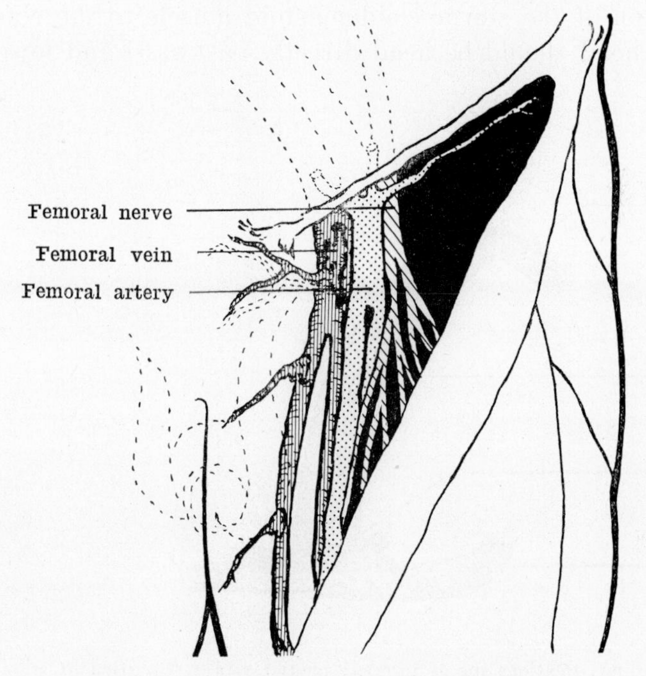

Fig. 19.—Anatomic relationships of femoral vein.

INTERNAL JUGULAR VEIN PUNCTURE—Cont'd

Certain anatomic relationships must be kept in mind. These are demonstrated in Figs. 20 and 21. It is well to point out that a study of the cross-section through the neck at the level of the clavicular heads (Fig. 21) reveals the proximity of the common carotid artery to the internal jugular vein. In addition, the apical portion of the lungs with pleura also is relatively close. For these reasons, special precaution must be taken during internal jugular venipuncture. The thrust of the needle should neither be too vigorous nor hasty. If a successful venipuncture is not made on the first trial, it is generally better not to probe blindly with the needle in the tissues. Only individuals with previous training should attempt to use this vein for routine venipuncture—except under unusual circumstances such as circulatory collapse. As can be seen in Fig. 22, the superficial site for the introduction of the needle should be at the angle formed with the clavicle by the insertion of the sterno-cleidomastoid muscle to the clavicle. The head should be head directly backward and lower

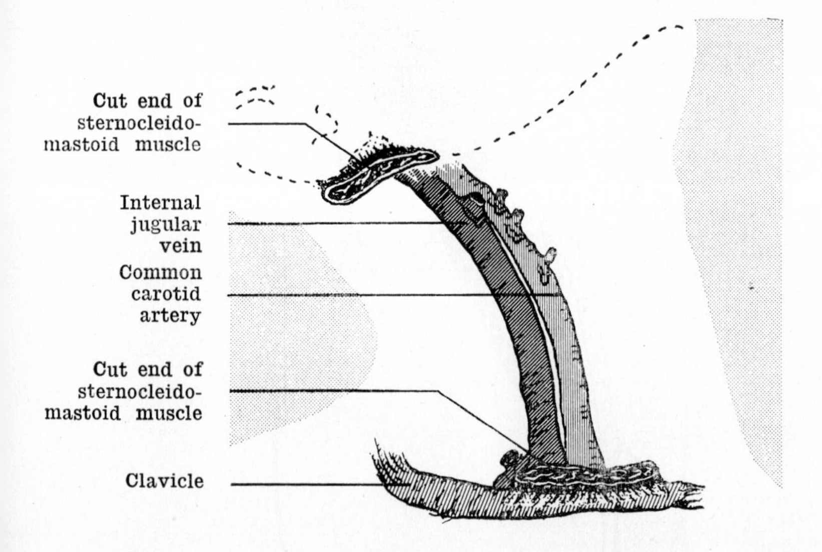

Fig. 20.—Anatomic relationships of internal jugular vein at insertion of sterno-cleidomastoid muscle to clavicle.

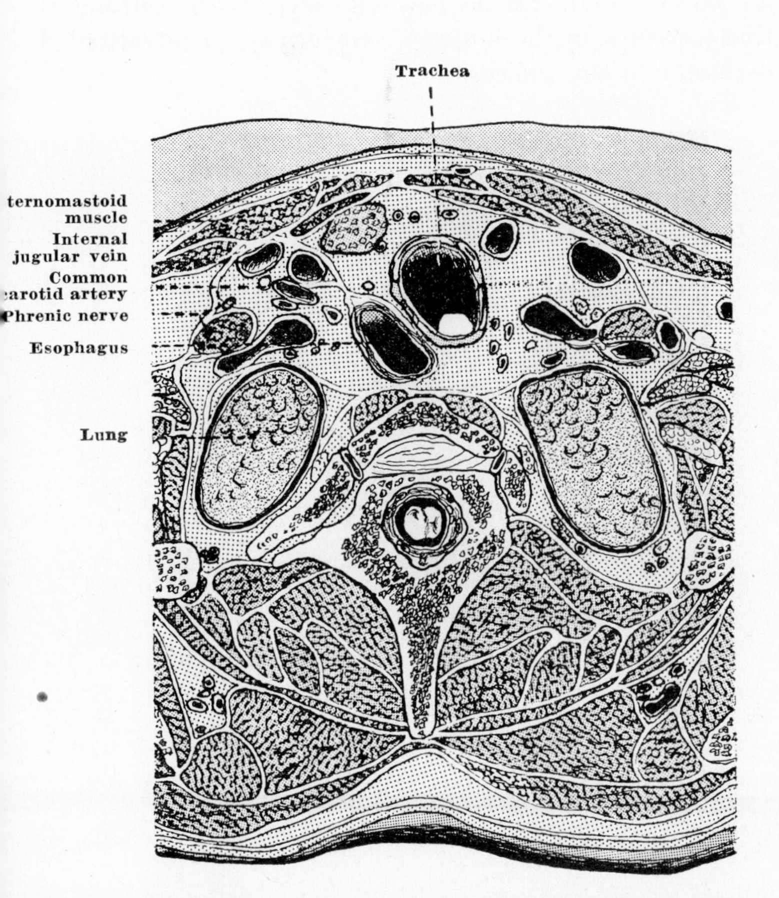

Fig. 21.—Cross section of neck at level of head of clavicle showing important anatomic relationships of internal jugular vein.

INTERNAL JUGULAR VEIN PUNCTURE—Cont'd

than the body. The needle should be directed toward the jugular notch—it should be pushed slowly with continuous negative pressure in the syringe. Generally, penetration of approximately 3 cm. suffices.

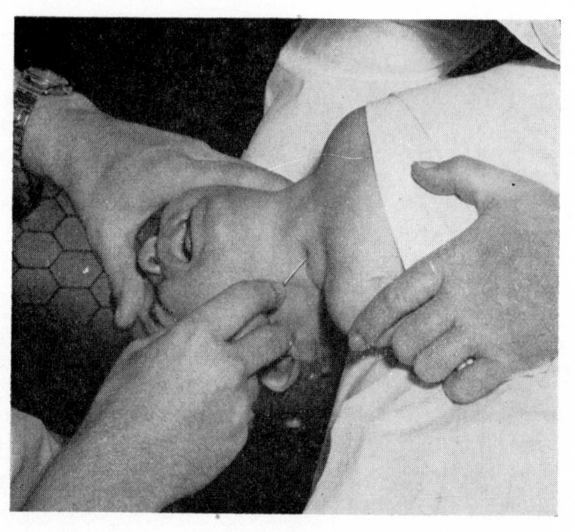

Fig. 22.—Position for puncture of internal jugular vein.

HAND VEIN PUNCTURE

It is not generally appreciated that the veins on the dorsum of the hand and on the volar aspect of the wrist are well suited for continuous intravenous therapy in infants and children. These vessels are small but easily accessible. Restraint may be achieved by the use of the arm board (Fig. 23) or a sandbag (not shown). The same general principles are applicable as in the case of cubital vein(s) puncture. For continuous intravenous therapy not only should the needle have a short bevel, but the needle should also be short (1 to 1¼ inch).

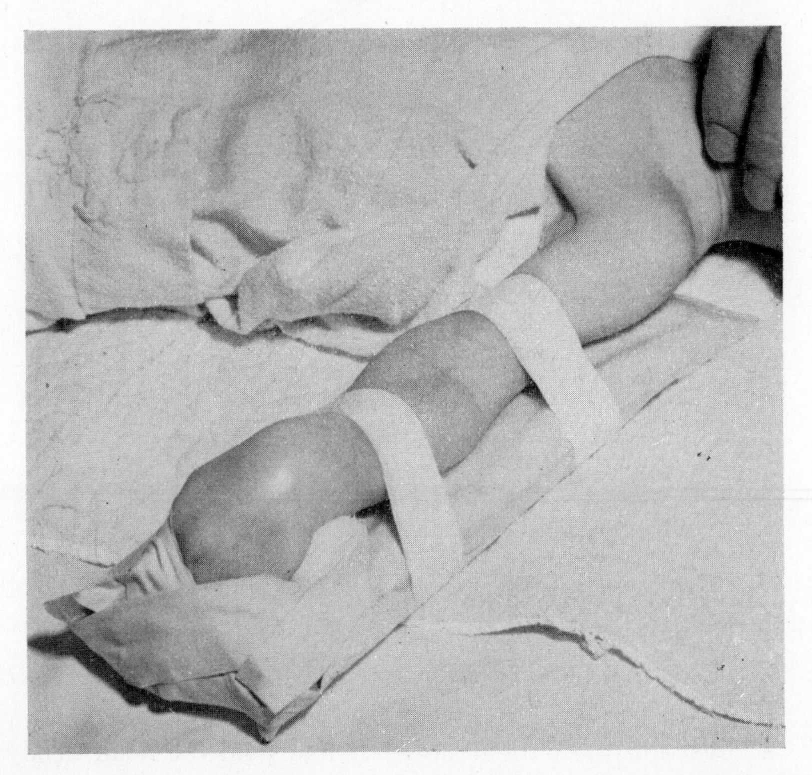

Fig. 23.—Proper restraint of upper extremity for venipuncture of hand vein.

SCALP VEIN PUNCTURE

Puncture of the scalp veins is most frequently done in infants. Occasionally, sufficient blood may be withdrawn from a scalp vein for diagnostic purposes. More frequently, however, scalp veins are used for the administration of intravenous fluids or medication. The vessels most frequently used are those indicated in Fig. 24. Other vessels, especially on the forehead, may occasionally be used. These vessels are generally adequately distended when the infant cries.

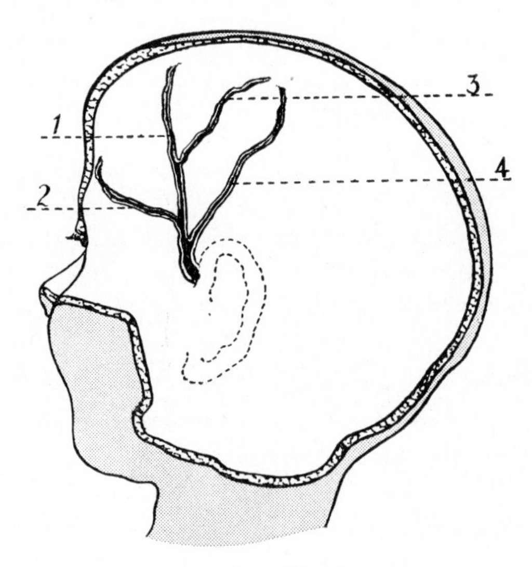

Fig. 24.—Anatomy of superficial temporal veins. *1, 2, 3,* and *4* are common tributaries of the superficial temporal vein.

1. Shave the area if necessary.
2. Prepare the skin aseptically.
3. Use a sharp, short-bevel, short (1 inch) No. 22 to No. 27 gauge needle.
4. Restrain the patient properly and hold the head firmly (Figs. 25 and 26). Although the method of restraint pictured here has proved valuable and practical in our experience, other workers have devised a variety of

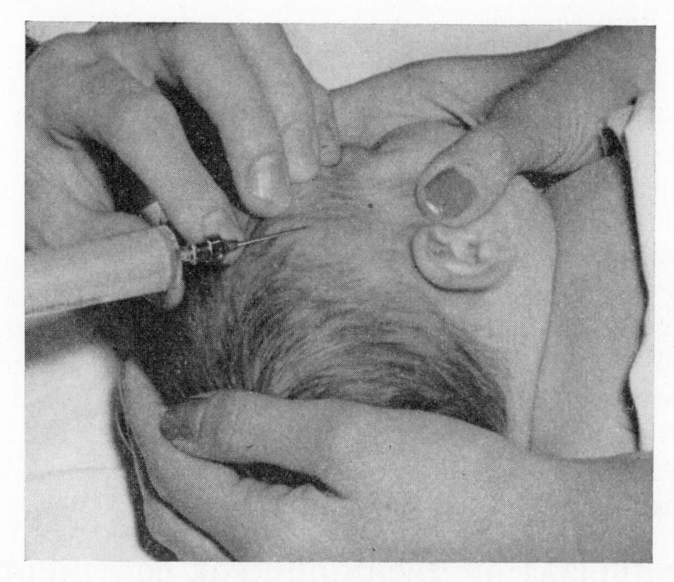

Fig. 25.—Scalp vein puncture.

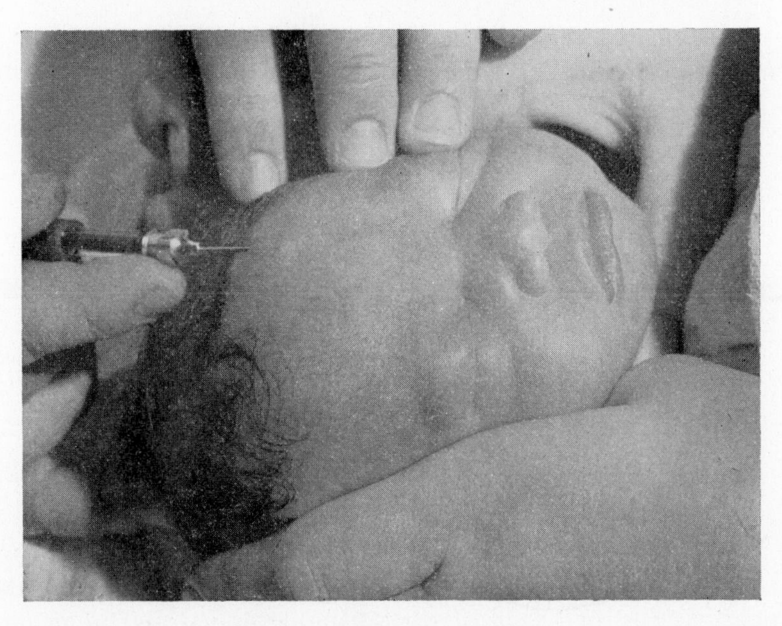

Fig. 26.—Scalp vein puncture.

SCALP VEIN PUNCTURE—Cont'd

mechanical restraints which require less personal assistance but also permit the use of these veins for continuous intravenous therapy. These mechanical devices include either a series of clamps or several sandbags. These methods are valuable whenever inadequate personnel is a real problem.

5. Puncture the skin over the vessel gently. The vessel usually is quite superficial. Thus, if the thrust is too vigorous, the deep wall of the vein will also be penetrated with subsequent hematoma formation.
6. Hold the needle firmly.
7. After removing the needle, exert pressure for several minutes at the site of venipuncture.

CANNULIZATION TECHNIQUE FOR CONTINUOUS INTRAVENOUS MEDICATION

Occasionally, difficulty is encountered in keeping an intravenous needle in place for continuous intravenous therapy in

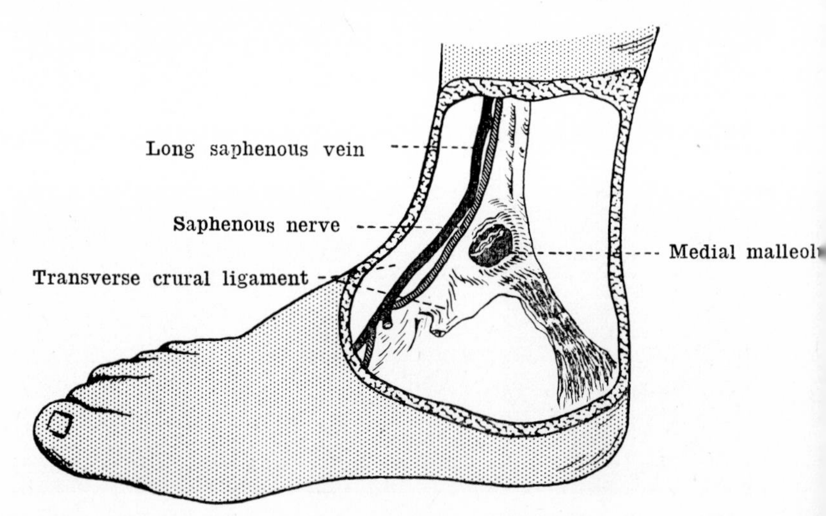

Fig. 27.—Anatomic relationships of great (long) saphenous vein at ankle.

CANNULIZATION TECHNIQUE FOR CONTINUOUS INTRAVENOUS MEDICATION—Cont'd

infants and children. Under such circumstances surgical exposure of the large saphenous vein at the ankle may be necessary in order to cannulate the vessel. The anatomic landmarks are shown in Fig. 27. The proper restraint for this procedure is demonstrated in Figs. 28, 29, and 30. Occasionally other suitable superficial vessels may be used for this purpose.

1. The proper surgical preparation of the skin should always be performed.
2. The operator should wear sterile rubber gloves.
3. A small area over the vein is infiltrated with 1% Novocain (Fig. 31).
4. An incision is made perpendicular to the vein and across the vein about ½ inch long (Fig. 32). This procedure should expose the subcutaneous tissue.
5. The vein should be identified and isolated by spreading the skin and subcutaneous tissues apart with a hemostat. (Fig. 33.)
6. Ligatures are placed around the vein but are not tied. (Fig. 34, *A*.)
7. A small incision is made into the vein.
8. A small blunt-end cannula* (18 to 22 gauge) is slipped into the vein and is tied with the ligature.
9. Sterile pads are used to dress the wound and properly to support the hub of the cannula, adaptor, and intravenous tubing. (Fig. 34, *B*.)
10. If the saphenous vein is used for this procedure, the leg should be examined frequently because thrombophlebitis may develop after 48 hours. Should evidence of this occur (as may be seen by red streaks along the course of the vessel in the leg), another vein should be selected.

*A polyethylene plastic catheter as recommended by Ingraham may be used in place of the usual metal cannula.

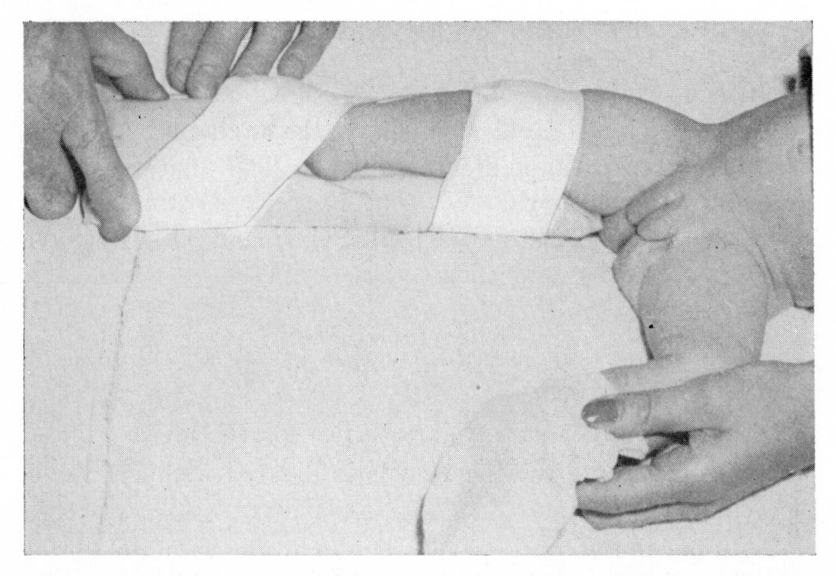

Fig. 28.—Proper restraint of leg for cannulization of long saphenous vein—Step 1.

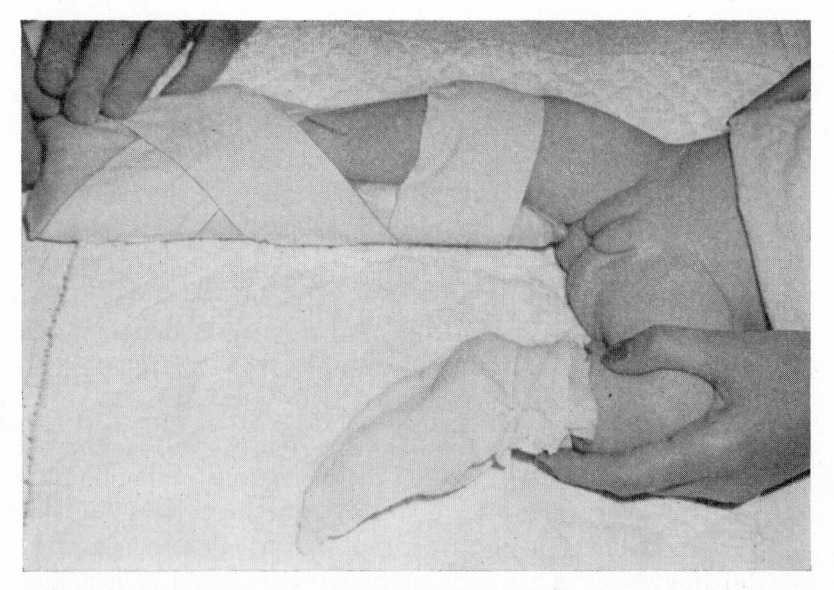

Fig. 29.—Proper restraint of leg for cannulization of long saphenous vein—Step 2.

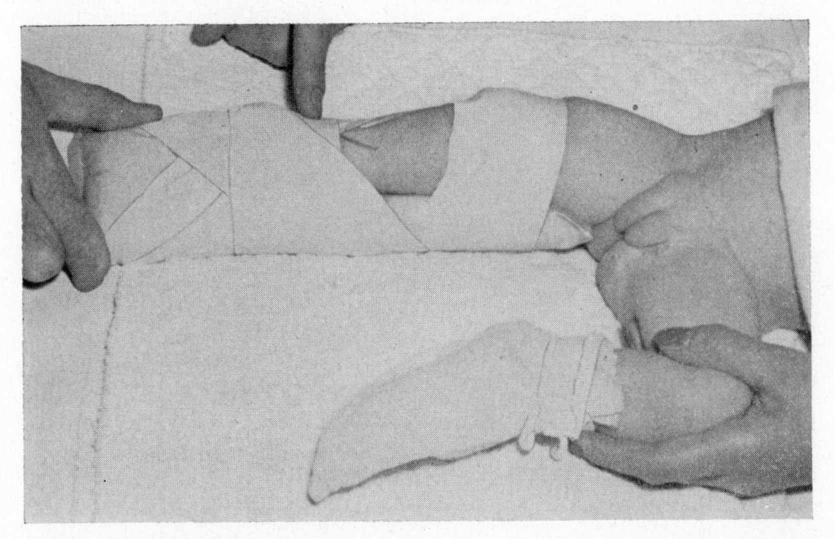

Fig. 30.—Proper restraint of leg for cannulization of long saphenous vein—Step 3.

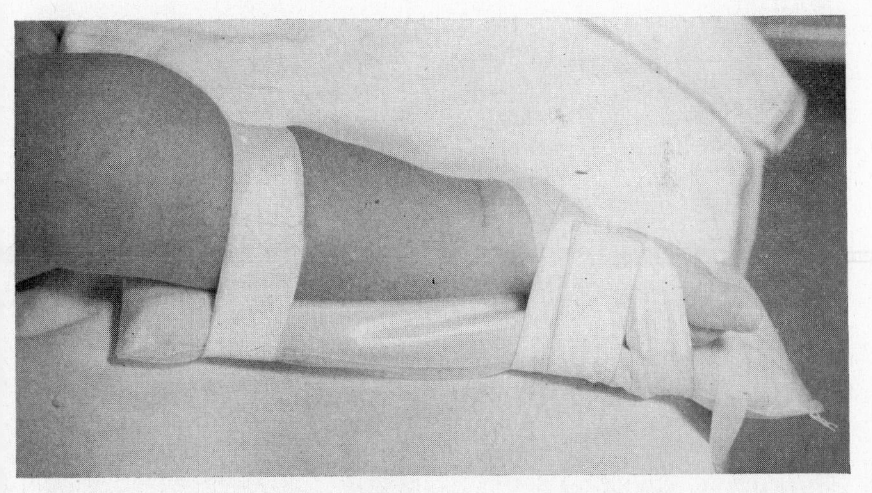

Fig. 31.—Proper restraint and site of incision for saphenous vein cannulization.

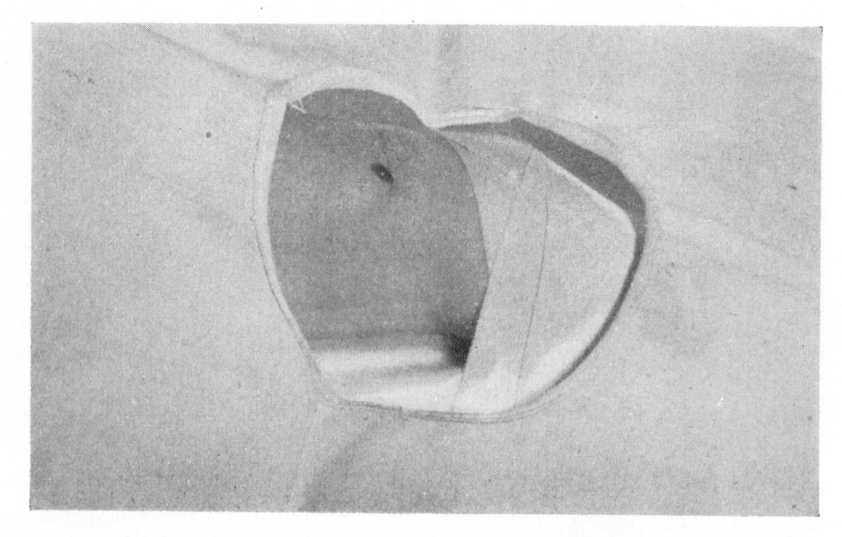

Fig. 32.—Incision of skin, perpendicular to vein.

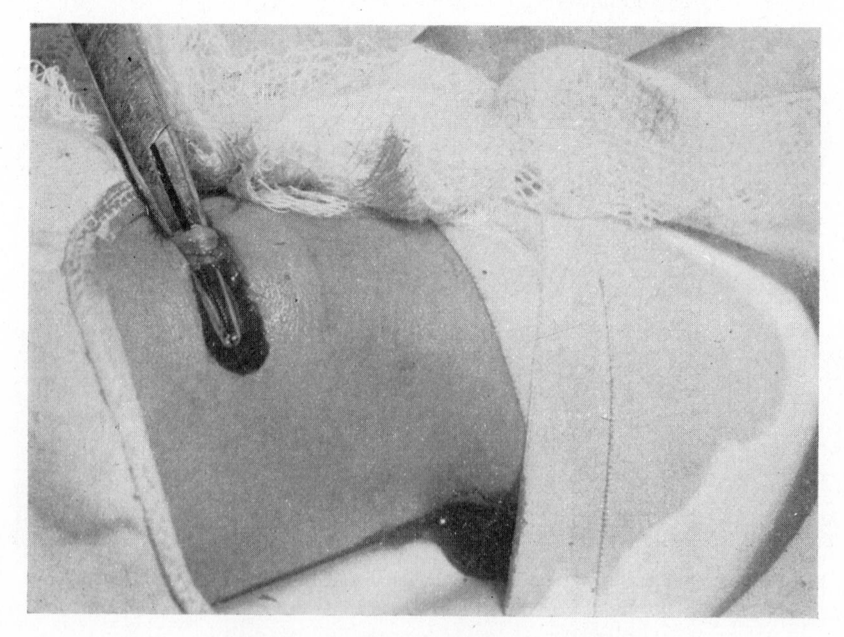

Fig. 33.—Exposing vein with hemostat.

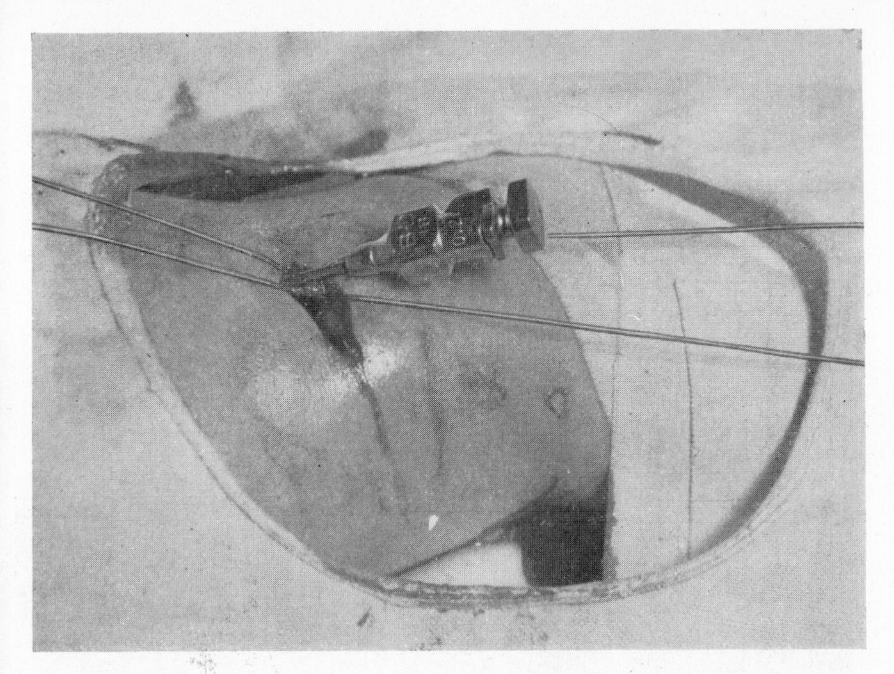

A.

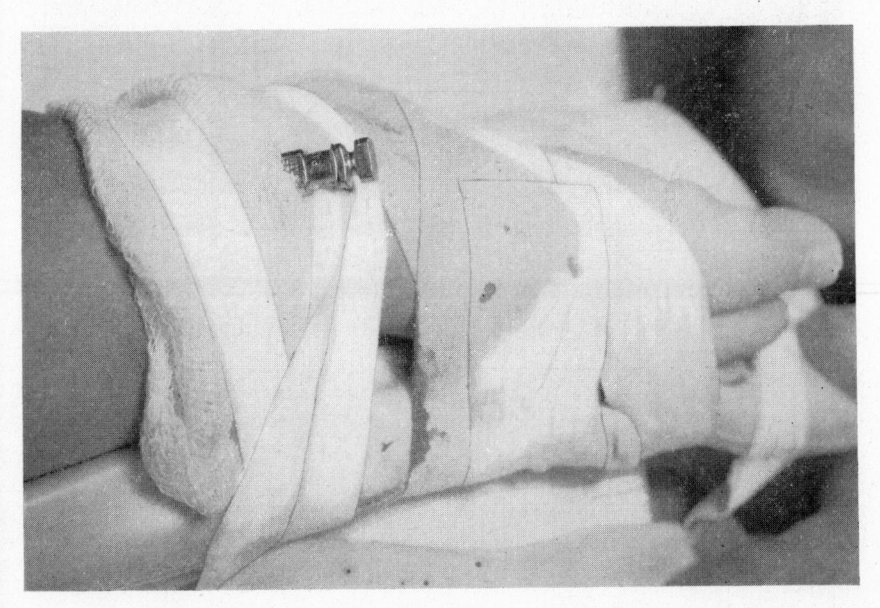

B.

Fig. 34.—*A,* Cannula in place with ligatures placed but not tied. One is drawn cephalad and one caudad to bring vein out superficially. *B,* Sterile pads for dressing and supporting the hub of the cannula, adaptor, and intravenous tubing.

HYPODERMOCLYSIS

A variety of fluids may be administered by this means to infants and children. These include physiologic saline, M/6 sodium lactate, Ringer's solution, hypotonic Ringer's solution, 2.5% dextrose in water or in physiologic saline, 1 to 5% solutions of sodium sulfadiazine, sulfamerazine, or combinations of these two sulfonamides.

Hyaluronidase may be used to hasten absorption of fluids given by hypodermoclysis (except when sulfonamides are being administered) as directed in another section (page 31).

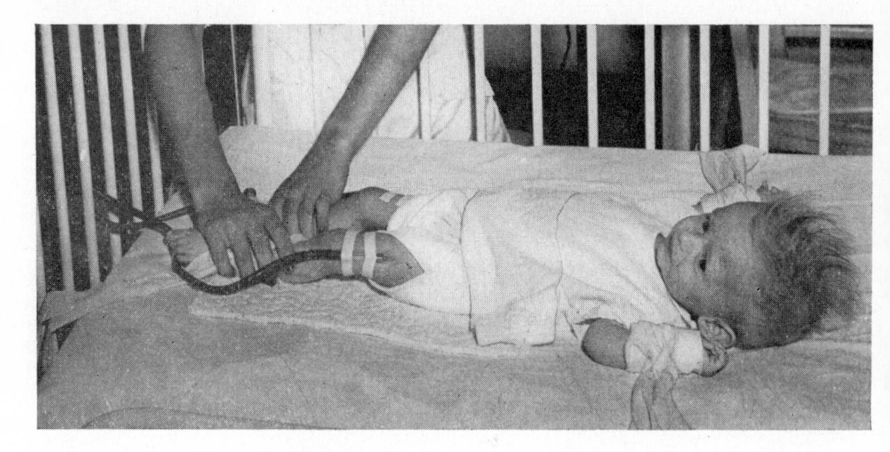

Fig. 35.—Restraint of patient for hypodermoclysis.

1. Proper restraint is required (Fig. 35).
2. The lateral aspects of the thighs are generally most suitable.
3. Proper asepsis is essential.
4. Number 22 gauge needles are inserted into a fold of skin picked up between two fingers.
5. The hub of the needles and the adaptor are secured by taping of the skin surface of the thighs.

VENOCLYSIS

This is a commonly used method for the administration of fluids and medications. Any available vein may be used.

For practical purposes, two methods may be differentiated: The constant drip method and the so-called rapid infusion or pump method. The advantages, disadvantages, and technique of each will be discussed.

CONSTANT DRIP VENOCLYSIS

Advantages

1. The necessary fluid and electrolytes to meet maintenance requirements may be administered gradually over a period of time.
2. One avoids overloading the circulatory system.
3. If untoward reaction occurs to the parenteral fluid or medication being administered, the administration may be interrupted either temporarily or completely.
4. The needle remains in place, allowing periodic intravenous administration of medications.

Disadvantages

1. Prolonged restraint of the patient is necessary.
2. The needle may gradually become loosened, either partially or completely thus allowing extravasation.

Technique

1. Perform venipuncture using appropriate vein.
2. Secure needle in place.
3. Adjust flow of fluid according to needs of patient.
4. Check rate of flow of fluids periodically.

RAPID INFUSION OR PUMP METHOD

Advantages

1. The patient need be restrained for a relatively short period of time.
2. It is easily performed in young infants.

VENOCLYSIS—Cont'd
RAPID INFUSION OR PUMP METHOD—Cont'd

Disadvantages

1. Too rapid infusion may precipitate cardiac failure in the debilitated infant.
2. Should an untoward reaction occur, a large amount of fluid or medication has already been injected.
3. Frequent venipunctures may be necessary if periodic fluid administration is essential.

Technique

1. A set-up as seen in Fig. 36 is generally necessary. This consists of:
   (a) A reservoir (in the illustration a bottle of blood is used for this purpose).
   (b) A drip bulb with filter attached to the reservoir.

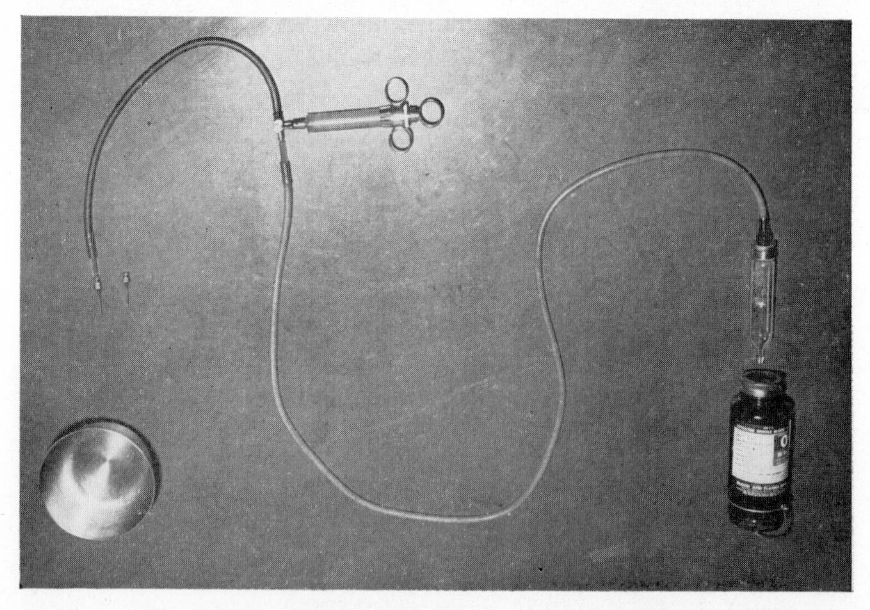

Fig. 36.—Practical arrangement for "pump" venoclysis.

VENOCLYSIS—Cont'd
RAPID INFUSION OR PUMP METHOD—Cont'd
Technique—Cont'd

(c) Rubber or plastic tubing, 4 to 5 feet long, attached to the drip bulb.
(d) A three-way stopcock attached to the opposite end of the rubber or plastic tubing.
(e) A 10 or 20 c.c. syringe attached to the central portion of the three-way stopcock.
(f) Another piece of rubber or plastic tubing (1 to 1½ feet long) attached to the third part of the three-way stopcock.
(g) A glass adaptor and proper needles attached to the other end of this second piece of tubing.
(h) A sterile basin containing sterile citrated isotonic saline.

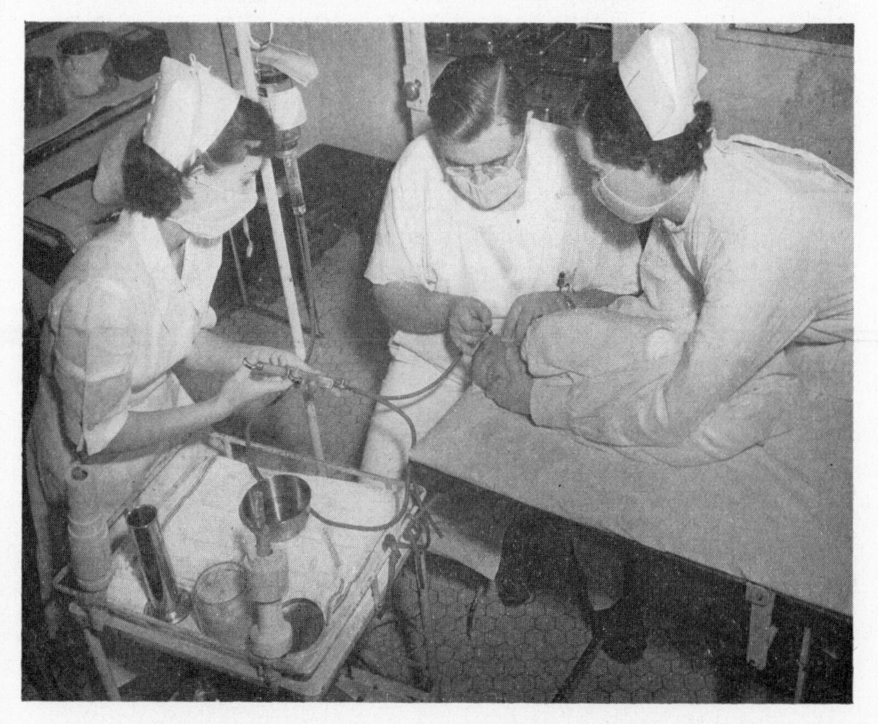

Fig. 37.—"Pump" venoclysis in a small infant. Restraint and technique.

VENOCLYSIS—Cont'd
RAPID INFUSION OR PUMP METHOD—Cont'd
Technique—Cont'd

2. Fill distal tubing and syringe with saline.
3. Fill tubing between three-way stopcock and reservoir bottle with fluid to be administered.
4. Perform venipuncture.
5. When needle is securely in the vein, expel saline from syringe into vein.
6. Fill syringe subsequently with fluid from reservoir by turning the three-way stopcock to proper position. (Fig. 37.)
7. Continue filling of syringe and expelling into vein (each time properly adjusting the stopcock positions).
8. Do not exceed 10 c.c. per minute in older children or 2 to 5 c.c. per minute in infants.
9. When pumping whole blood or concentrated red blood cells, rinse syringe frequently with sterile, citrated, isotonic saline to prevent "freezing" of the plunger in the barrel of the syringe.
10. Have 1 or 2 spare sterile syringes available should a technical difficulty arise.
11. Observe the patient carefully for any ill effects—especially pallor, cyanosis, dyspnea, nausea, excessive perspiration, urticaria, or fever. Stop procedure at once should any of these symptoms or signs develop.

GASTRIC LAVAGE

This procedure may be used in both infants and older children. Generally the oral route may be used for the introduction of the tube in infants, whereas the nasal route is frequently easier in older children. A No. 8 to No. 10 French catheter is applicable for infants, while a small Levine tube or a No. 10 to No. 12 French catheter may be used in older children. The length of the tubing which must be passed is generally equivalent to the distance from the nasal bridge to the tip of the xiphoid process.

GASTRIC LAVAGE—Cont'd

1. Restrain patient.
2. The head must be held firmly and turned to one side.
3. Pass a cooled, moistened catheter or tube gently through the mouth (in infants) or nose (in older children) into the esophagus and then into the stomach.
4. Generally speaking, if the trachea is entered, severe coughing and dyspena will be induced.
5. Attach a bulb syringe and introduce lavage fluid. Withdraw fluid through tube. If an obstruction occurs to flow at this time, attempt to expel material into the stomach and try again.
6. Save all lavaged material in cases of suspected poisoning.
7. Always close the tube by pinching before withdrawing from the stomach.

LUMBAR PUNCTURE

This procedure may be done for diagnostic or therapeutic purposes. The positions generally used for adults should be used. Certain points bear emphasis.

1. Strict asepsis is mandatory.
2. Excellent restraint is of real aid. This is especially true when the puncture is acutely made. Sudden motion of the patient at this moment may cause a traumatic tap.
3. The equipment shown in Fig. 38 is generally adequate.
4. The third or fourth lumbar interspace is generally chosen.
5. The spinal needle should be introduced slowly to avoid striking the wall of the canal with its associated blood vessels.
6. The spinal fluid should be examined as directed on page 57.
7. A sterile dressing should be applied to the puncture site after the tap.

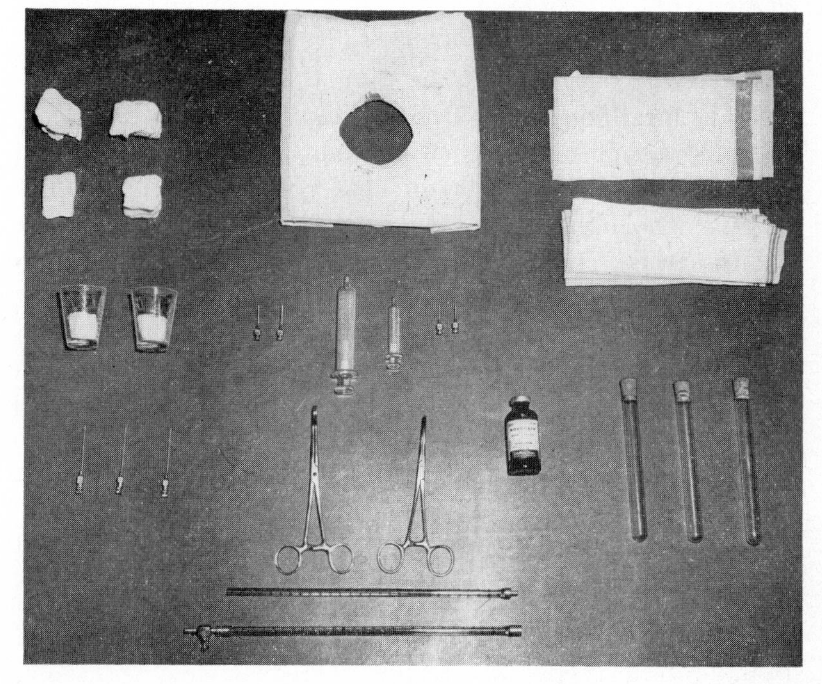

Fig. 38.—Equipment for lumbar or subdural puncture.

SUBDURAL TAP

Technique

1. Sedate the infant if necessary and restrain properly. (Fig. 39.)
2. Strict asepsis is of utmost importance.
3. The head should be shaved widely—at least 2 inches posterior to the anterior fontanel, 2 to 4 inches lateral to the midline and forward to the forehead.
4. The head should be immobilized by the nurse.
5. The area is prepared with either iodine and alcohol or tincture of Merthiolate and sterile gloves and towels are used. (Figs. 40 and 41).
6. The lateral margins of the anterior fontanel are palpated along the coronal suture and a site 2-3 cm. from the midline is chosen. (Fig. 42.)

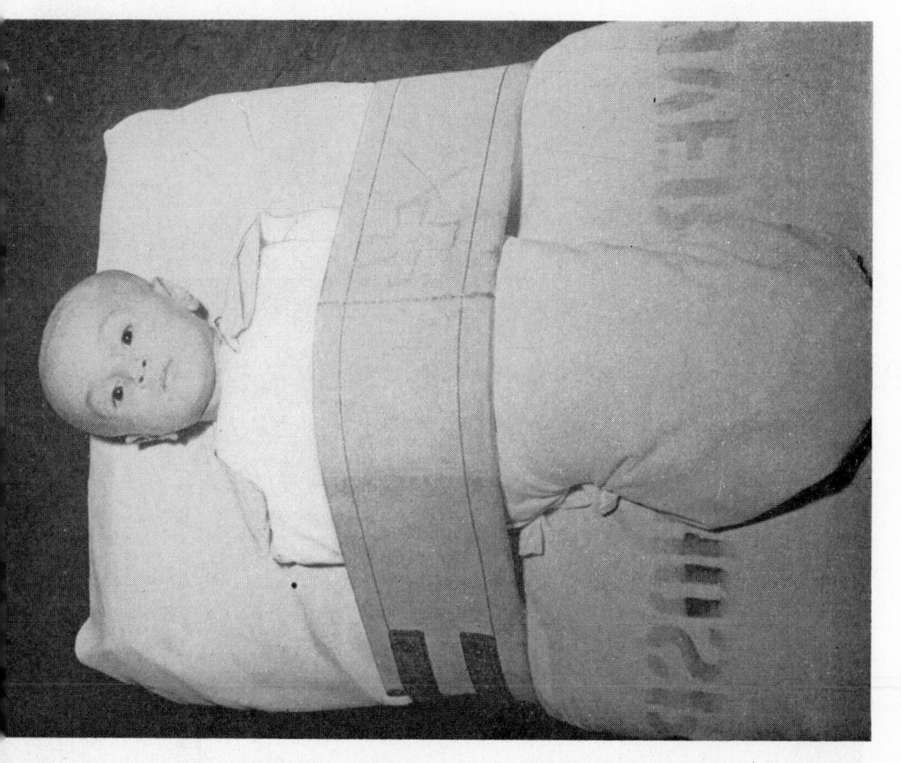

Fig. 39.—Body restraint for subdural puncture.

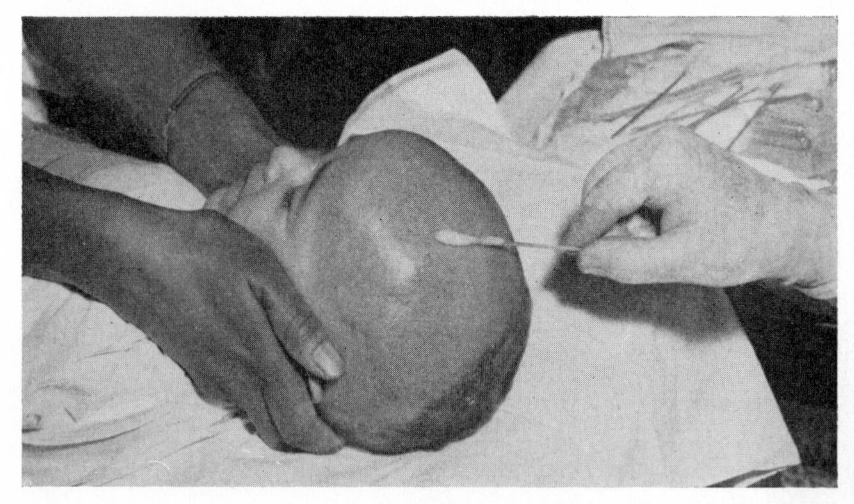

Fig. 40.—Preparation for subdural puncture, including proper immobilization of head.

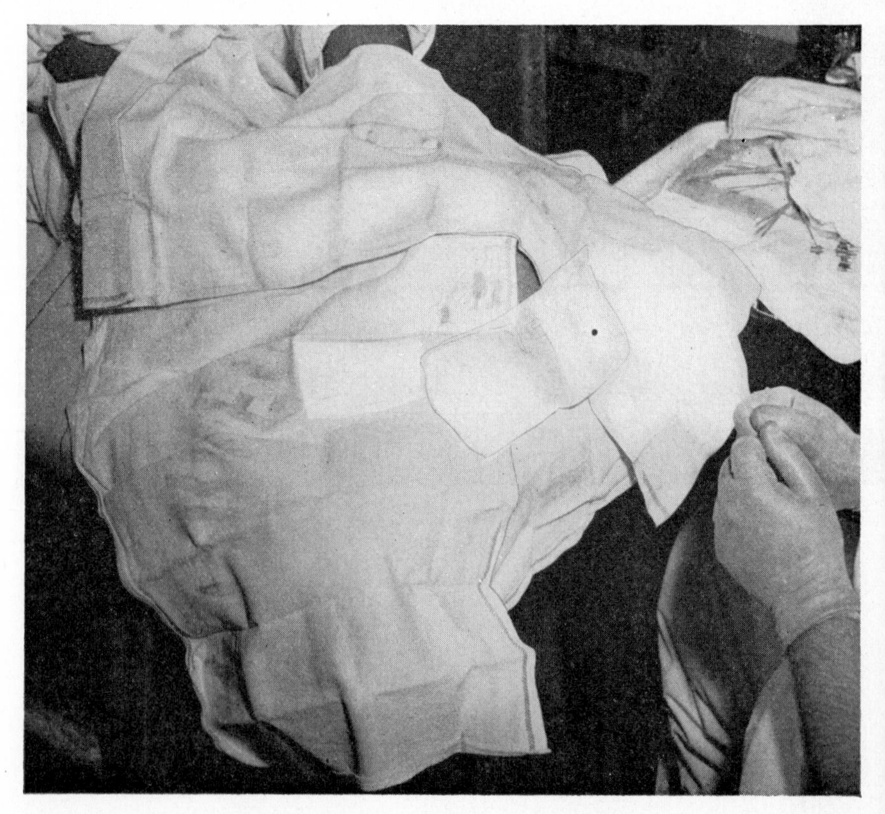

Fig. 41.—Sterile towels are properly placed.

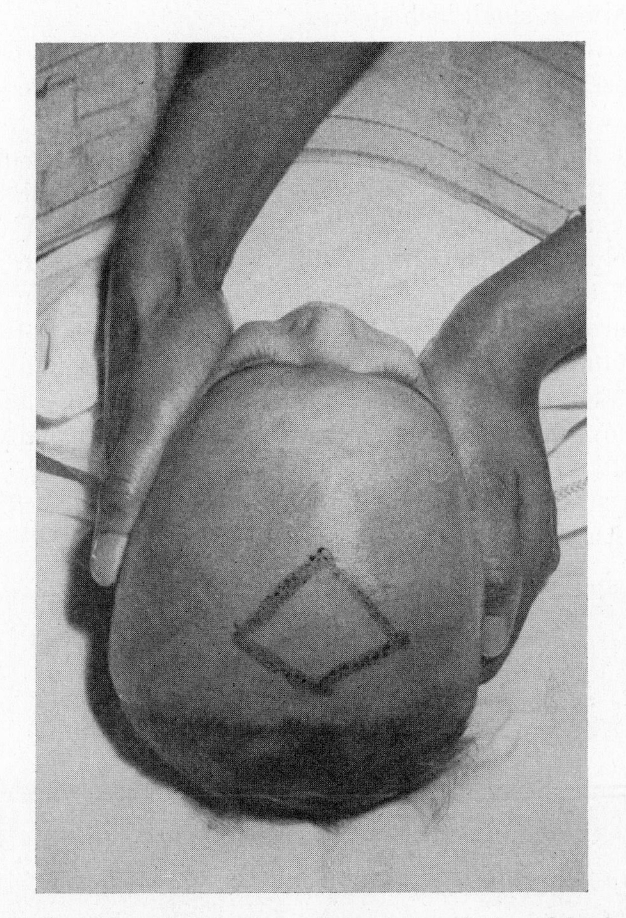

Fig. 42.—Outline of margins of anterior fontanel as guide for subdural puncture.

SUBDURAL TAP—Cont'd
Technique—Cont'd

7. The skin over the puncture site is injected with 1% Novocain—a small bleb suffices.
8. A No. 20 short-bevel spinal puncture needle is carefully inserted at right angles to the scalp into the skin, through the suture line, and into the subdural space, to the depth of approximately ⅛ to ¼ inch. (Fig. 43.) A puncture is performed on both sides in a similar manner. On a negative tap no fluid or only a few drops of a clear, colorless fluid will be obtained with a protein content of 15-30 mg.%. Abnormal fluid may either be xanthochromic or grossly bloody; the latter does not clot on standing. In most instances the abnormal fluid will be under increased pressure and 10 to 15 c.c. can be removed; the protein content of this fluid is usually markedly elevated.
9. A sterile gauze dressing should be tightly affixed. (Fig. 44.)

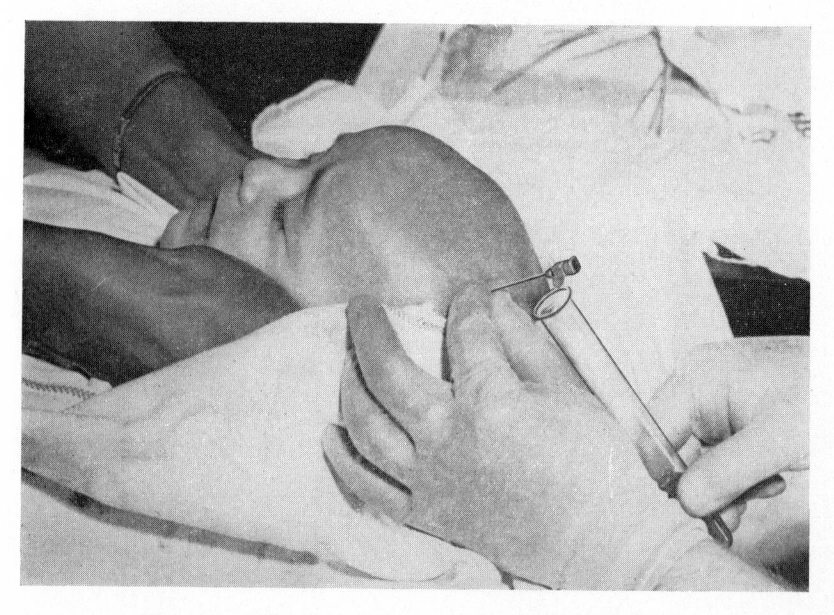

Fig. 43.—Collection of fluid from subdural hematoma.

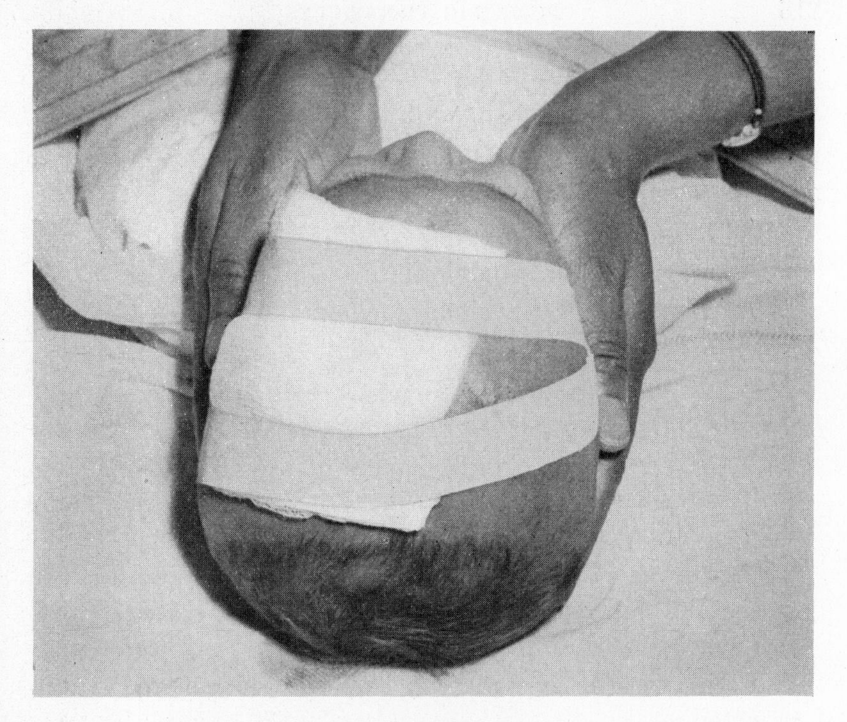

Fig. 44.—Dressing in place after subdural puncture.

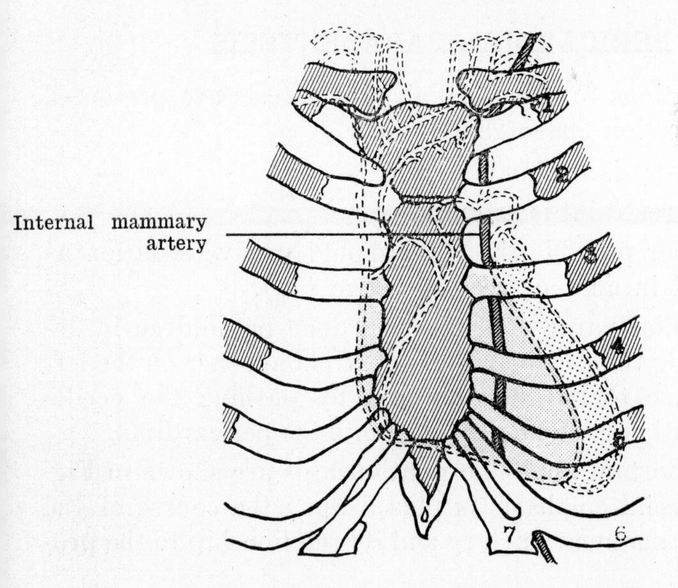

Fig. 45.—Important anatomic relationship for pericardial paracentesis.

ABDOMINAL PARACENTESIS

This procedure is occasionally performed as an emergency procedure to relieve embarrassment to respiration due to marked ascites in children with the nephrotic syndrome. Certain points bear emphasis.

1. Strict asepsis is mandatory.
2. Always empty the bladder completely by catheterization.
3. Avoid midline punctures.
4. The child should be in a sitting position.
5. A tight abdominal binder should be used to avoid sudden hypotension crisis following the removal of large amounts of fluid.
6. Preoperative administration of sedation (as outlined in section on Preanesthetic Medications, page 176) is frequently useful to allay apprehension.
7. Local anesthesia with 1% Novocain is generally indicated.

PERICARDIAL PARACENTESIS

The indications for pericardial paracentesis are presented in another section (page 23).

1. Strict asepsis is mandatory.
2. Proper restraint is essential.
3. Whenever possible the child should receive sedation as outlined in another section (page 176).
4. Pericardial paracentesis is best done in children by introducing the needle in the costoxiphoid space on the left side close to the sternum and by pushing the needle backward and slightly upward into the pericardium.
5. The important anatomic relationships are shown in Fig. 45. Special emphasis is placed upon the course of the internal mammary artery and its relationship to the procedure.

TRACHEOTOMY

Occasionally, tracheotomy must be performed as an emergency procedure. Whenever possible, an airway should be used as a guide. Frequently, however, this is not possible. The anatomic landmarks are presented on Fig. 46.

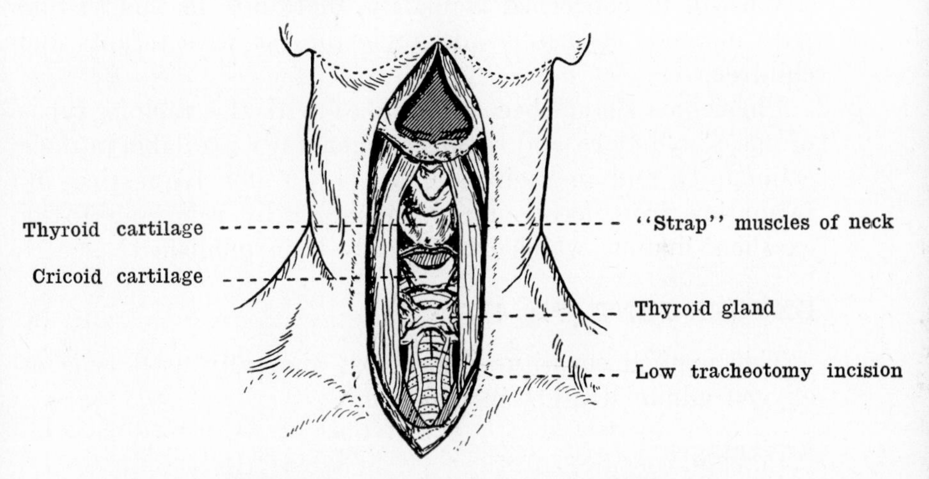

Fig. 46.—Important anatomic landmarks in tracheotomy.

1. Observe asepsis if possible.
2. Make an incision about 2 to 3 cm. long from above the thyroid isthmus downward. Separate the muscles exposed.
3. Stop bleeding by sponging (or hemostats, if available).
4. Incise 3 tracheal cartilaginous rings in the midline.
5. Insert tracheotomy tube.
6. Secure with taps around the neck.
7. Apply sterile dressings to the open parts of the wound.
8. Maintain patency of tracheotomy tube by frequent cleansing.

OXYGEN THERAPY

The fundamental principles of oxygen therapy and especially the practical application of these principles may fre-

OXYGEN THERAPY—Cont'd

quently play an important part in emergency care of patients. There is really little need to emphasize the all-important role which oxygen plays in the management of a variety of disorders.

We will be concerned primarily, therefore, in this section with methods especially adaptable for use with infants and children.

Physicians should become familiar with the various types of gases, cylinders, and regulators generally available in their community and in their hospitals by either requesting information from local supply houses or by referring to an excellent manual which has recently been published.[1]

OXYGEN TENT (Fig. 47)

This method constitutes the most generally used type of oxygen administration in children.

Advantages

1. Best suited for children because it is comfortable as soon as they overcome fear of the setup.
2. Best suited for oxygen therapy which must be prolonged.

Disadvantages

1. There is an extra demand on nursing aid.
2. The initial cost is high.
3. Oxygen concentrations are very variable, depending upon frequency and duration of other treatments which necessitate opening of the tent.
4. Maximum oxygen concentration is 60%—under optimal conditions.

Special Instructions and Precautions

1. The temperature should be at approximately 68° F. for children (higher for newborn infants; i.e., the same as nursery temperature).

OXYGEN THERAPY—Cont'd
OXYGEN TENT—Cont'd
Special Instructions and Precautions—Cont'd

2. Humidity of 35 to 50% should be maintained.
3. Oxygen flow should be 6 to 10 liters per minute. This generally maintains a concentration of approximately 50% oxygen within the tent.
4. In order to bring oxygen concentration back to optimum concentration after opening the tent, flood the tent with oxygen at 12 to 14 liters per minute for about 3 minutes.
5. The oxygen flow should never fall below 4 liters per minute.

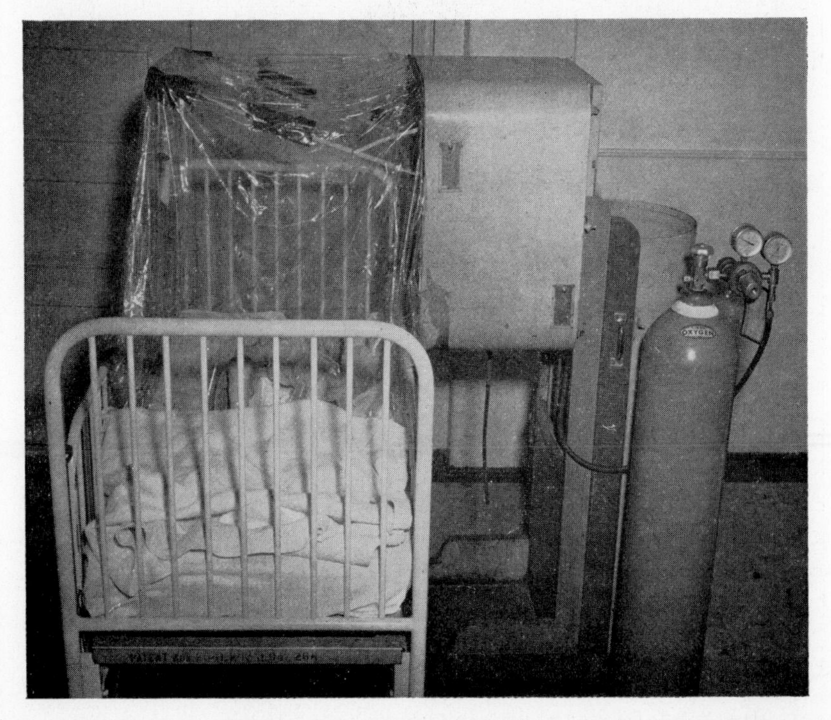

Fig. 47.—Oxygen tent with cooling and humidifying device between oxygen source and canopy.

OXYGEN THERAPY—Cont'd

OPEN TOP OXYGEN TENT (Fig. 48)

This method is primarily intended for infants and small children.

Advantages

1. Less expensive and more easily stored than regular oxygen tent.

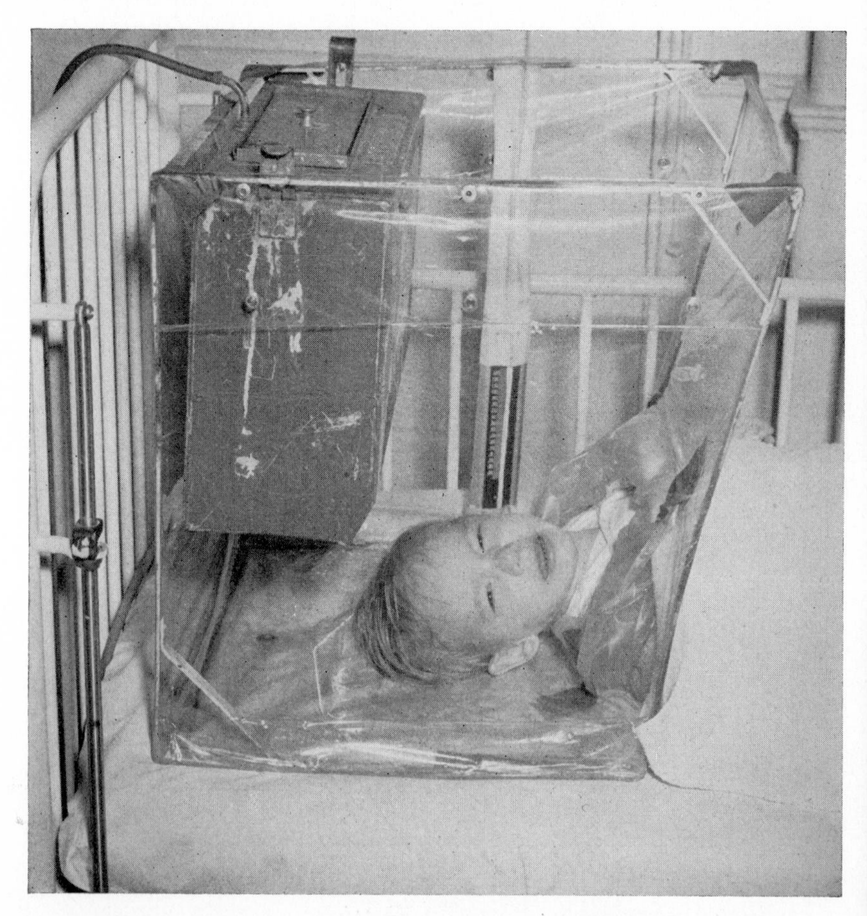

Fig. 48.—Open top tent showing compactness and small ice unit.

OXYGEN THERAPY—Cont'd
OPEN TAP OXYGEN TENT—Cont'd
Advantages—Cont'd

2. May be used on smallest crib in nursery.
3. Oxygen concentrations obtained are those obtained with regular oxygen tent.
4. Higher oxygen concentrations (up to 80%) may be obtained by increasing oxygen flow and closing top of tent.
5. Helium oxygen mixtures may be administered with this method.

Disadvantages

1. Cooling must be optimum so that oxygen should settle in lower part of tent.
2. Low oxygen concentrations may result from drafts in the room (and over open top), restlessness of patient, loose neck band, or hyperpnea.

Special Instructions and Precautions

1. Keep ice-cooling mechanism full all the time.
2. Oxygen flow should be 6 to 10 liters per minute.
3. Avoid smoking or open flame near tent.

OROPHARYNGEAL CATHETER

Occasionally this method becomes necessary to supplement the oxygen tent method or to replace it because of either claustrophobia or insufficient oxygen. It must be emphasized that this method differs from nasopharyngeal placement. The tip of the catheter should be in the oropharynx. While this is frequently difficult to manage and maintain in children, nasopharyngeal placement generally replaces oxygen concentration by about 10%.

Advantages

1. Simplicity.
2. Requires minimal nursing care.
3. Inexpensive.

Disadvantages

1. Should not be used in presence of acute or chronic nasal inflammation or nasal allergy.
2. Small children and infants may require arm restraints.
3. It may prove irritating.
4. Catheter may have to be cleansed and replaced frequently.

Special Instructions and Precautions

1. Use No. 8, No. 10, or No. 12 French oxygen catheters, depending on size of patient.
2. Oxygen flow should be 2 to 6 liters per minute.

AEROSOL THERAPY

This form of combined oxygen and antibiotic therapy has great usefulness in pediatrics. One of three methods is generally used by us.

Special Hood (For Infants) (Fig. 49)

As can be seen from Fig. 49, this consists of a small metal frame (9 × 7½ × 7½ inches) covered with transparent plastic. The hood is placed over the head and closed by means of a drawstring mechanism. The aerosol tube is attached to an oxygen source. Both penicillin and streptomycin may be aerosolized in this way. Oxygen should flow at a rate of 6 to 8 liters per minute and generally the amount of solution used can be completely aerolized in about 3 to 5 minutes.

This method is not to be used for children over 2 years of age because the space within the hood is so small that high concentration of CO_2 may accumulate within the hood with older children.

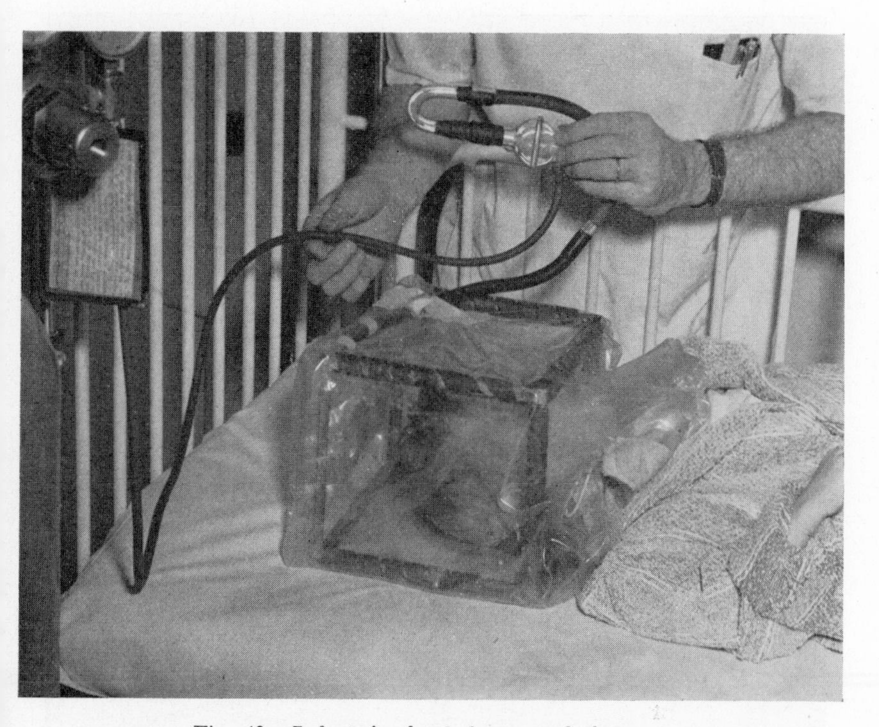

Fig. 49.—Infant-size hood for aerosol therapy.

AEROSOL THERAPY—Cont'd

Barach or Boothby Mask (For Older Children) (Fig. 50)

This method can be used for children over 2 years of age. The same principles pertain as outlined in Special Hood method on page 222.

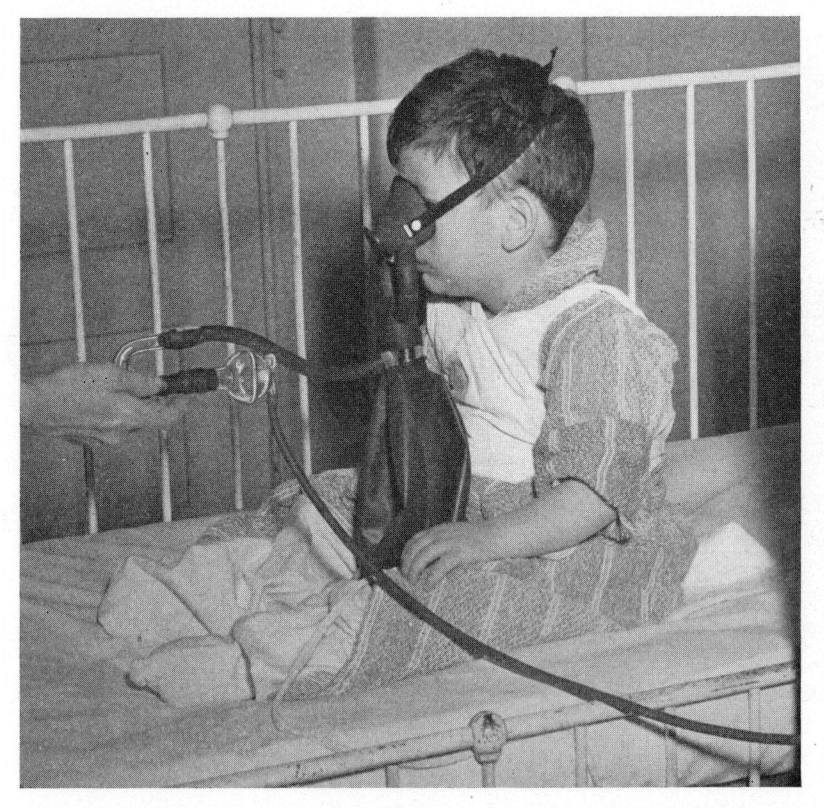

Fig. 50.—Mask for aerosol therapy in older children (only for nasal use).

AEROSOL THERAPY—Cont'd

Croupette (For Infants and Older Children Also) (Fig. 51)

This device is extremely useful whenever high concentrations of oxygen and moisture are necessary in therapy. This type of apparatus is available commercially.

The accompanying figure shows the essential points. A small opening is present to permit attachment of an aerosol tube.

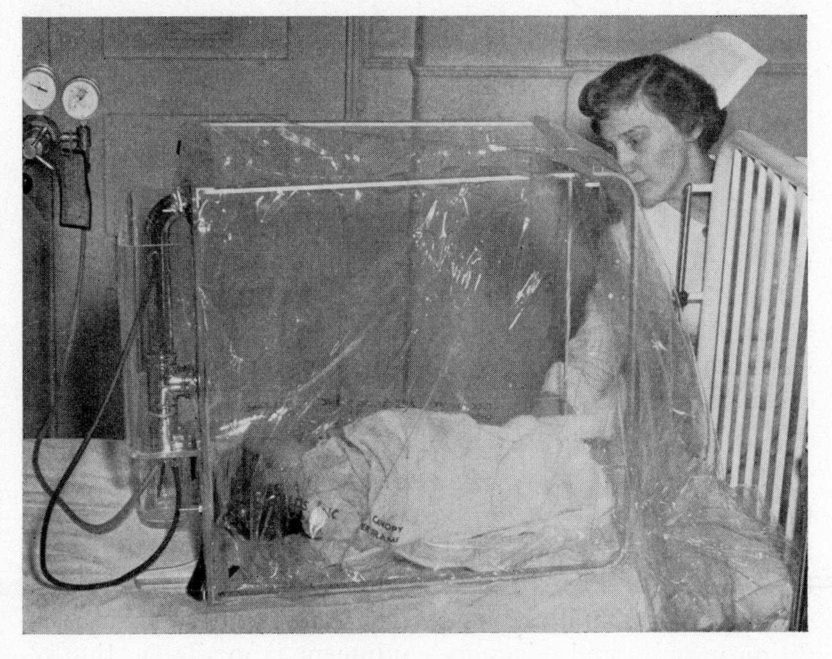

Fig. 51.—Croupette.

Reference

1. Andrews, A. H., Jr.: Manual of Oxygen Therapy Techniques, Chicago, 1947, The Year Book Publishers, Inc.

ADDENDA*

CHAPTER IV

MANAGEMENT OF ACUTE HEAD INJURIES[1] (See also page 53)

Recently,[1] certain features in the management of acute head injuries have been presented through the cooperation of neurologists and neurosurgeons. Originally prepared for a bulletin for the Committee on Trauma of the American College of Surgeons, it was reprinted in a recent journal.[1] It is presented herewith in slightly modified form to supplement the material in the text.†

Head injuries may be classified as open and closed. Open injuries incur the risks of (1) hemorrhage and (2) wound infection. Closed injuries involve the risks associated with (1) immediate destruction of brain tissue (contusion, laceration, etc.), and (2) progressive damage secondary to (a) cerebral compression due to intracranial hemorrhage or edema and (b) anoxia resulting from an inadequate airway.

For clarity, the treatment of open and closed wounds will be considered separately in this paper, but it is to be emphasized that both often are seen in the same patient and require consideration jointly.

Treatment of Open Wounds

The proper treatment of lacerations of the scalp consists of thorough cleansing, débridement, and snug closure. As a first-aid measure, a compression bandage should be applied to control bleeding. Externally protruding foreign bodies should not be manipulated. When the patient's general condition permits and adequate equipment is available, the following procedure should be undertaken:

1. Shave scalp widely about the wound.
2. Cleanse wound with soap and water and irrigate thoroughly with copious amounts of solution (saline or water).

---

*These articles were prepared after the main text had been completed. The chapter numbers listed refer to the original chapters in which each article actually belongs.

†This material, from this point to the end of paragraph F on page 231, was originally prepared by a special committee of the Harvey Cushing Society.

3. Infiltrate margins of scalp wound with procaine.
4. Remove dirt and excise devitalized portion of scalp.
5. Explore skull for fracture.
6. If no fracture, close wound snugly in one or two layers with interrupted sutures of nonabsorbable material.
7. Give antitetanic serum or tetanus toxoid.

Simple lacerations may be closed in the emergency room by a single operator, but it is more satisfactory if the operator has an assistant to compress the margins of the wound to control bleeding.

Where the laceration overlies a fracture, surgical correction should be undertaken only in the operating room, for it may be necessary to remove dirt, hair, or debris from the fracture line or to remove bone fragments. One should be prepared to deal with bleeding from the dura and brain.

If the brain is lacerated or foreign bodies are retained within the brain substance, all macerated brain tissues should be removed, the foreign bodies removed if possible, particularly if they are nonmetallic, all bleeding controlled, and the dura and scalp closed snugly. Surgical treatment of these wounds requires experience in brain surgery and special equipment (suction, lighting, electrocoagulation, etc.). With the use of chemotherapeutic and antibiotic agents, it is permissible to defer operative closure of wounds for many hours pending improvement in the patient's general condition and analysis of his neurological status.

Leakage of cerebrospinal fluid from the nose or ear constitutes a special problem. Any cerebrospinal fluid fistula invites the risk of meningitis. Now, with an adequate screen of antibiotic and chemotherapeutic agents, one is justified in waiting ten to twelve days pending spontaneous closure. If the leak persists longer than this, surgical closure of the fistula should be considered. Some feel that lowering of the spinal fluid pressure to 90 mm. of water by spinal drainage every twelve hours promotes spontaneous closure. Fortunately most fistulas do close spontaneously.

Closed Wounds

One of the most frequent causes of death after head injury is progressive cerebral damage due to anoxia. Many factors contribute to this:

1. The capacity of the contused brain to utilize oxygen is diminished.
2. The cerebral blood flow is reduced, even though blood pressure may be elevated.
3. The oxygen concentration of the blood is diminished as the result of a disturbed respiratory center and obstruction of the respiratory tract (tongue, mucus, pneumonitis).

The treatment in such cases is the maintenance of an adequate airway and the administration of oxygen. Patients frequently improve remarkably after clearing the airway and administering oxygen. The most satisfactory way of giving oxygen is by nasal catheter. Oxygen tents and masks interfere with attempts to keep the airway patent. Constant nursing attention, with a suction apparatus for the removal of mucus, is necessary. This may be supplemened by postural drainage (head down on face). Tracheotomy is indicated in certain cases.

The differential diagnosis between surgical and nonsurgical lesions is of primary importance in the management of acute head injuries and usually depends upon the patient's course. Hence, a carefully taken history, particularly as relates to the onset and duration of unconsciousness, and frequent and repeated neurological examinations are necessary.

Intracranial clot, such as extradural, subdural, or intracerebral hematoma, usually is incompatible with life and requires surgical removal. Most patients with these lesions show progressive stupor, convulsions, focal paralyses, and disturbance of the vital signs, such as alteration in pulse, respirations, etc. If the patient has been conscious and then loses consciousness, an expanding intracranial lesion is probably present. The lucid interval may be prolonged (days or weeks) with subdural hematoma. If the patient has remained continuously unconscious from the moment of impact, the coma may be due in part to contusion of the brain and in part to an expanding lesion. In such instances, it may be impossible to make a differential diagnosis clinically, and cranial exploration then is necessary if the patient's condition is growing worse.

The surgical management of these lesions is not within the scope of this book.

Special Examinations and Treatments

A. *X-rays.*

X-rays of the skull rarely influence the course of treatment yet the procedure of taking films involves considerable manipulation and wastes time, both of which are detrimental to the ill patient. Hence, it is advisable that x-ray examination of the skull be deferred until such time as the patient is cooperative and his condition stabilized. Attention should always be given to the possibility of injury elsewhere, particularly to the cervical spine.

B. *Position of Patient.*

The position of election is with the head elevated, since this reduces venous congestion. The advantages of this position, however, are far outweighed by the disadvantages which might accrue from an obstructed airway, and if the patient's airway cannot be kept completely open with the head elevated, this position should be changed to one which best promotes an adequate airway.

C. *Shock.*

Surgical shock (peripheral vascular collapse) is rare in head injuries per se, but, when present, the usual measures (Trendelenburg position), intravenous fluids, etc.), should be employed. Shock usually indicates associated injuries and demands primary consideration.

D. *Fluid Balance.*

In an effort to reduce or limit cerebral swelling after head trauma, certain writers have advocated rigid dehydration by withholding fluids, administration of hypertonic solutions intravenously, the use of magnesium sulfate enemas, etc. Rigid dehydration does harm rather than good to an ill patient, as the other vital body functions are interfered with.

It is necessary in this connection to keep close watch upon the protein metabolism. Coma, stupor, and prolonged confusion often result from protein depletion and can be prevented or corrected by the administration of protein hydrolysates, plasma, or whole blood. If coma is prolonged, gastric feedings by nasal catheter are indicated, using a high protein diet.

E. *Spinal Puncture.*

Considerable controversy prevails concerning the indications for and the merit of spinal puncture in the diagnosis and treatment of head injuries. Some advocate daily spinal punctures as routine in the treatment of head injuries, but this is not generally accepted. The authors (of the original article) consider the indiscriminate use of spinal punctures dangerous. The following are considered proper indications for spinal puncture.

1. Diagnostic.
   (a) To determine pressure where intracranial clot is suspected.
   (b) To determine the presence and/or degree of bleeding.
2. Therapeutic.
   (a) To lessen intracranial pressure by withdrawing fluid as a temporary expedient pending measures that provide more lasting control of increased intracranial tension, such as surgical evacuation of clot.
   (b) Evacuation of bloody fluid when signs of meningisimus appear, usually four to eight days. Evacuation of fluid at this time usually relieves headache and speeds recovery.

Technique.

When indicated, a spinal puncture should be done with the patient in the lateral recumbent position, using a standard spinal puncture needle.

The operator should make the following determinations: color of the fluid, initial pressure, final pressure and the amount withdrawn.

Jugular compression tests should not be carried out unless one suspects injury to the spinal column. These tests give no information of value with reference to the brain, and the sudden rise in spinal fluid pressure which follows jugular compression may be harmful after head injury.

Spinal puncture should not be attempted if the patient is uncooperative, for the information obtained is unreliable, and struggling against resistance may be harmful.

F. *Control of Restlessness.*

Patients who are restless and confused constitute a difficult nursing problem, and sedative medication may be necessary. Paraldehyde administered rectally or barbiturates—Sodium amytal, Luminal sodium—intramuscularly or intravenously are satisfactory. The latter are particularly indicated for the control of convulsions. Morphine and codeine are contraindicated because of depression of respirations, edema of the larynx, and alteration of pupils (diagnostic).

CHAPTER IV

Bacitracin therapy for staphylococcic meningitis (See also page 66).

The therapy of staphylococcic meningitis has been quite successfully managed with penicillin, sulfa, and the antibiotics listed in the chapter. Nevertheless, occasionally resistance will develop to all of these agents. Recently[1a, 1b] the antibiotic bacitracin has been administered successfully in several such cases. Naturally, optimum dosage schedules and methods of administration remain to be established. Nevertheless, a tentative schema applicable to infants is presented:

(1) *Bacitracin intramuscularly.* 400 units per kilogram every 6 hours for 4 days. Then, 200 units per kilogram every 6 hours for one more week.

(2) *Bacitracin intrathecally.* 500 units in 3.0 c.c. isotonic saline twice daily for 4 days. Then, same dose once daily for one more week.

One must recall too, however, that the earliest reports of systemic bacitracin administration indicated (as with polymyxin) a nephrotoxicity. This should be looked for and, if serious, therapy interrupted.

CHAPTER IV

Coma in Diabetes Mellitus (See also page 70)

The problem of management of patients in diabetic coma remains a complex one. As has been previously stated, "routine orders" to take care of all such patients are definitely to be discouraged. A fine quantitative and qualitative assessment of the needs of the individual patient—both from the laboratory (including EKG) and clinical viewpoint—is constantly essential; of course, excellent supervision is mandatory.

Many different parenteral fluids have been suggested—as also in the management of diarrhea. The detailed and analytical approach of Butler[2] and co-workers merits attention and inclusion here. Although the hypotonic Ringer's solution used by Hartmann (see pages 30 and 71) contains potassium, apparently an increase of potassium in therapy seems indicated from the available, recent evidence.

General Procedure

1. Stimulate renal function and re-establish normal circulation by the administration of an appropriate saline-lactate or saline-bicarbonate solution.* Such a solution should be given in quantities of 800 ml. per square meter of body surface† at a rate of 8.0 ml. (140 drops) per square meter per minute. The total amount should be administered in about 1 to 2 hours.
2. In accordance with the needs of the patient as determined by the hemoglobin, hematocrit, and/or serum proteins, a transfusion of 300 ml. per square meter of body surface should be given.
3. A hypotonic, multiple electrolyte solution‡ should be then started if the circulation and renal function are satisfactory. The rate should be 3 ml. (50 drops) per square meter per minute.
4. When nausea is eliminated, the remainder of the parenteral solution may be given orally.

One must emphasize, however, that the administration of potassium intravenously or even subcutaneously may lead to toxicity. Thus, repeated, frequent EKG and serum potassium levels are essential. Furthermore one must be well trained in the interpretation of these EKG's because in these may be the earliest signs of potassium intoxication. The EKG changes associated with potassium intoxication are as follows:

1. Increase in the height of the T waves with a sharpening of the contour of the T waves.

*400 c.c. isotonic saline, 40 c.c. Molar Na Lactate, 560 c.c. distilled water.

†See Appendix, Table III, for chart showing measurements of square meter body surface.

‡Hypotonic, multiple electrolyte solution
(a) Concentrations per liter:
Na,53 mEq.; Cl,45 mEq.; K,25 mEq.; mg.5 mEq.; P, 0.2 Gm.
(b) Preparation:
To one liter of 5-10% glucose in distilled water add:
2.8 Gm. Na lactate
1.8 Gm. Na Cl
1.0 Gm. KCl
1.0 Gm. K_2HPO_4
0.3 Gm. $MgCl_2$§
0.15 Gm. $NaH_2PO_4 \cdot H_2O$
(pH 7.4)

§Autoclave $MgCl_2$ separately and add separately. All other constituents may be autoclaved together and kept sterile in small vials.

2. A broadening of the QRS complex with loss of the ordinary contours.
3. Changes in the S-T and T segments.
4. Disappearance of the P wave.

CHAPTER IV

Terramycin.

This newest of the available antibiotic agents is effective against a variety of pathogens (comparable in spectrum to aureomycin). Preparations for oral as well as intravenous administration are available. Although no optimum dosage schedule is available, approximately 100 mg. per kilogram is the suggested one in infants. Older children should receive 1 to 2 Gm. daily.*

Intravenous therapy.

1. Dilution of intravenous preparation:

   Contents of one 250 mg. ampule in at least 100 ml. diluent.
2. Precautions must be taken to prevent extravasation.
3. Terramycin should be administered slowly intravenously (10-20 drops per minute).
4. Multiple sites for intravenous administration should be chosen.

CHAPTER V

Care of Patients With Bulbar Poliomyelitis (See also page 93)

Increasing research in the pathologic physiology of patients with bulbar poliomyelitis has lead to the concept of electrophrenic respiration[3, 3a] in the management of these patients. It is quite clear from available statistics that the mortality and morbidity in bulbar poliomyelitis has been and is high. Accordingly, one must utilize all available methods in the attack on this problem. The method of electrophrenic respiration offers such an approach. Neither the technique

*The oral route is most commonly used.

nor the theory of the method is to be presented, but the physician should be aware of the fact that patients may be carried over a very critical period with this method of therapy.

CHAPTER V

MEDIASTINAL EMPHYSEMA

Recent experience with this problem made us feel that it merited its inclusion. To be sure, the more serious forms are less common than the forms in which only a small amount of air may be seen in the mediastinum on x-ray. A brief review of contributing factors may aid in the analysis of symptoms, signs, and treatment. These are in accordance with the concepts of Hamman[4] and others.[5, 6, 7]

Contributing Factors

Primarily interstitial pulmonary emphysema resulting from

(1) Spontaneous alveolar rupture.
(2) Thoracic trauma.
(3) Increase of intrapulmonary pressure.

Symptoms and Signs

(1) Pain, mild to severe.
(2) Subcutaneous or retroperitoneal emphysema.
(3) Obliteration of cardiac dullness.
(4) Peculiar sounds over heart.
(5) Evidence of increased mediastinal pressure.
(a) Cyanosis, (b) dyspnea, (c) engorged veins, (d) circulatory failure.
(6) Pneumothorax
(7) X-ray evidence.

Treatment

(1) General supportive therapy only necessary in mild cases.
(2) Surgical consultation for mediastinotomy in more severe cases.

CHAPTER VII

Poisoning Due to Drugs (See also page 134)

Management of patients with poisoning due to the following drugs was inadvertently omitted from the main text:

ACONITE

1. Avoid general emetics.
2. Lavage promptly with plain water.
3. Follow with lavage with 1:1000 to 1:10,000 potassium permanganate.
4. Follow treatment of acetanilid poisoning (page 138).

AMINOPHYLLINE

Occasionally, a marked idiosyncrasy results in toxicity to even small quantities of aminophylline, especially when given too rapidly intravenously.

Symptoms are generally those of circulatory collapse.

Treat as outlined in section on shock (page 182).

CARBON MONOXIDE POISONING

Poisoning with this agent is only too frequent. Although therapy as outlined in the main part of the text is generally of value, an additional method has been presented[7a] in the use of intravenous procaine hydrochloride. The dose and method of administration are presented on page 178.

DICHLORICIDE AND DICHLORPHENOL

Treat as outlined under benzene derivatives (page 138).

ETHYL ALCOHOL

Not infrequently, children ingest various ethyl alcohol preparations. All degrees of central nervous system effects have been encountered and recorded. These varied from inebriation (CNS—cortical inhibition) to deep stupor (CNS depression).

Treatment

1. Keep patient warm.
2. *Avoid apomorphine.*

3. Lavage with water.
4. Use caffeine sodium benzoate, ephedrine, Metrazol, or Coramine as outlined in section on barbiturate poisoning (page 135).
5. Antibiotics to control secondary pulmonary infection.

FLUOROACETATE (COMPOUND 1080)

This highly toxic agent is being used widely at present as a rodenticide.

Toxicity and Symptoms and Signs

1. CNS—convulsions.
2. Cardiovascular—arrhythmias, heart failure.

Treatment

1. Highly unsatisfactory but experimentally ethyl alcohol seems to be an antidote.

IRON

In addition to the material in the text, the following suggestions have been made:

1. Produce emesis.
2. Lavage with aqueous sodium bicarbonate to convert the corrosive ferrous sulfate into the less irritating carbonate salt.

MAGNESIUM SULFATE

Intoxication due to this agent may result from its use as a cathartic or enema or when used parenterally in therapy of hypertensive encephalopathy. The latter may develop most readily in patients with extremely poor renal function.

Symptoms and Signs

1. Feeling of flushing.
2. Abdominal pain and distention.
3. Nausea.
4. Vomiting.
5. Shallow, irregular respirations.

6. Precipitous fall in blood pressure.
7. General flaccidity.
8. Bradycardia.

Treatment

1. Intravenous calcium therapy as outlined on page 38.
2. Artificial respiration until normal rhythm is re-established.
3. Adequate oxygen supply.

METHYL ALCOHOL

1. Recent evidence indicates that in the treatment of this problem the administration of ethyl alcohol may prevent methanol metabolism.

PHOSPHORIC ACID ESTERS (THIOPHOS, T.E.P., AND RELATED INSECTICIDES)[7b, 7c]

1. The symptoms and signs are those of physostigmine (see Mecholyl Poisoning).
2. Treatment as for mecholyl poisoning.

SALICYLATE INTOXICATION[8a]

1. Since dehydration is not usually a part of the picture when the poisoning has been accidental, M/3 sodium lactate may be given rather than the more dilute M/6.
2. Both ascorbic acid and vitamin K should be given early parenterally.

ZINC STEARATE

Poisoning resulting from inhalation of baby powders containing zinc stearate has become relatively uncommon. However, it may still be encountered in certain areas.

Symptoms and Signs

1. Marked coughing and dyspnea.
2. Numerous moist and musical râles throughout the lung fields.
3. Marked stridor.

4. Fever.
5. Cyanosis.
6. Choking.

Treatment

1. Oxygen in high concentrations.
2. Clean all powder from respiratory tree. Bronchoscopic aspiration may be indicated in the severe cases.
3. High humidity atmosphere as in laryngotracheobronchitis (page 83).
4. Antibiotics to prevent and/or control infection.

CHAPTER IX

BEE STINGS (See also page 154)

Two additional agents are of value in the symptomatic management of bee stings and also in the management of the anaphylactic shock response.

1. Subcutaneous epinephrine—in doses as for asthma (page 86).
2. Intravenous calcium gluconate as in tetany (page 34).

CHAPTER IX

SERUM REACTIONS (See also page 177)

Certain features, including suggested dosages for different age groups, should be emphasized.[9]

1. Always skin test patient with 0.1% procaine hydrochloride for sensitivity.
2. Administer intravenous procaine slowly (20-30 drops per minute). Although optimum dosages have not been established, the following is considered safe:

   (a) 2-5 years of age 125 to 250 c.c.
   (b) 5-10 years of age 250 to 500 c.c.
   (c) 10-15 years of age 500 to 750 c.c.

TABLE XIII. OBSERVATIONS OF VALUE IN FOLLOWING PATIENTS WITH HEMORRHAGE, TRAUMATIC SHOCK, BURNS AND OTHER BODY FLUID AND ELECTROLYTE DISTURBANCES

(From Janeway et al.: M. Clin. North America, 1945.[10])

OBSERVATIONS	METHOD	SIGNIFICANCE	
		HIGH VALUES	LOW VALUES
		A. Laboratory Data	
Hemoglobin or hematocrit	Hemoglobin Hematocrit reading Whole blood specific gravity	Hemoconcentration due to loss of plasma (Due to dehydration if total protein elevated)	Anemia due to red cell deficit or excessive plasma or saline
Total protein	Serum or plasma specific gravity	Hemoconcentration due to dehydration Hyperproteinemia	Hypoproteinemia due to plasma protein deficit or excessive saline
Chloride	Serum chloride	Renal disturbance Excessive saline Excessive CO_2 loss through lungs	Renal disturbance Excessive glucose solution Adrenal insufficiency Alkalosis
CO_2	CO_2 combining power of serum or blood	Alkalosis	Acidosis
Nonprotein nitrogen	N.P.N. or B.U.N. of serum or blood	Renal failure	Adequate renal function
Urine volume	12 or 24 hour collection	Satisfactory renal function—adequate renal circulation and proper fluid and electrolyte balance	Renal failure due to shock, dehydration, or actual renal disease
Urine specific gravity	Specific gravity	Dehydration	Normal response to water administration
		B. Clinical Data	
Skin temperature of extremities	Feel hands and feet	Warm = good peripheral circulation	Clammy, cold = poor peripheral circulation
Hydration of skin	Pinch skin, examine tongue, feel eyeballs	Soft and elastic skin = adequate hydration	Skin loose and dry = dehydration
Pulse	Pulse rate and quality	Rapid, feeble—shock	Slow, full—normal
Blood pressure	B.P. recorded regularly	High = increased intracranial pressure	Low = shock
Peripheral edema	Pitting of skin	If present, indicates adequate or excessive saline and ? low serum protein	
Pulmonary edema	Auscultation	If present = pulmonary injury (burns) or excessive blood, plasma, or saline	

3. Have Sodium amytal available for intravenous use in the event of excessive central nervous system stimulation; ephedrine sulfate is of value if circulatory collapse develops.

CHAPTER IX

SHOCK (See also page 180)

In addition to the material on burns, hemorrhage, and shock which is presented in Chapter IX, it was felt that a summary, quick-reference-type table might be of value in following patients with these problems. Such a table (Table XIII) has been presented by Janeway and collaborators[10] and is offered here as a practical guide.

References

1. Review Article: Management of Acute Head Injuries, New York Medicine, July 20, 1950.
1a. Teng, P., and Meleney, F. L.: The Treatment of Staphylococcic Meningitis, Surgery **28**: 516, 1950.
1b. Meleney, F. L., et al.: The Efficacy and Safety of the Systemic Administration of Bacitracin on Various Types of Surgical and Certain Medical Infections With an Analysis of 270 Cases, Surg., Gynec. & Obst. **89**: 657, 1949.
2. Butler, A. M.: Parenteral Therapy in Diabetic Coma, Acta paediat. **38**: 59, 1949.
3. Sarnoff, S. J., et al.: Electrophrenic Respiration in Acute Bulbar Poliomyelitis, J. A. M. A. **143**: 1383, 1950.
3a. Whittenberger, J. L., and Sarnoff, S. J.: Physiologic Principles in the Treatment of Respiratory Failure, M. Clin. North America **34**: 1335, 1950.
4. Hamman, L.: Mediastinal Emphysema, J. A. M. A. **128**: 1, 1945.
5. Macklin, M. T., and Macklin, C. C.: Malignant Interstitial Emphysema of Lungs and Mediastinum as Important Occult Complication in Many Respiratory Diseases and Other Conditions: Interpretation of Clinical Literature in Light of Laboratory Experiment, Medicine **23**: 281, 1944.
6. Aisner, M., and Franco, J. E.: Mediastinal Emphysema, New England J. Med. **241**: 818, 1949.
7. Abramson, H., et al.: Acute Pulmonary Interstitial and Mediastinal Emphysema (Airblock) and Pneumothorax in Infancy and Early Childhood, J. Pediat. **36**: 774, 1950.
7a. Olsen, C. W., et al.: Intravenous Procaine Hydrochloride in the Treatment of Asphyxia Due to Carbon Monoxide, Bull. Los Angeles Neurol. Soc. **14**: 23, 1949.
7b. Walker, J. T.: Toxicology, New England J. Med. **242**: 58, 1950.
7c. Grab, D.: Pharmacology and Toxicology of Certain Organic Phosphorus Insecticides, J. A. M. A. **144**: 105, 1950.
8. Thomson, J.: Ferrous Sulfate Poisoning; Its Incidence, Symptomatology, Treatment, and Prevention, Brit. M. J. **4654**: 645, 1950.
8a. Danielson, W. H.: Salicylate Intoxication, Bull. Child. Hosp. of Denver **1**: 172, 1948.
8b. Koszalka, M. F.: Hemoglobinuria in Bee Sting, Bull. U. S. Army Med. Dept. **9**: 212, 1949.
9. Schrum, D.: Intravenous Procaine in Children, J. Pediat. **34**: 433, 1949.
10. Janeway, C. A., et al.: Indications and Uses of Blood, Blood Derivatives, and Blood Substitutes, M. Clin. North America **29**: 1069, 1945.

APPENDIX

Appendix Table I. Commercial Sources of Poisons*

ABS Pills	Atropine	(134)	
	Strychnine	(142)	
ABSC Pills	Atropine	(134)	
	Strychnine	(142)	
Absorbine Jr.	Thymol	(131)	see Phenol
	Iodine	(128)	
	Menthol	(141)	see Salicylates
Acme Aphis Spray	Nicotine	(130)	
Acme Bait-M	Arsenic	(122)	
Acme Bordeaux Mix	Copper Sulfate	(142)	see Zinc Sulfate
Acme Duradust	DDT	(126)	
Acme Dura Spray	DDT	(126)	
Acme Paris Green	Arsenic	(122)	
Acme Red River Potato Mix	DDT	(126)	
	Arsenic	(122)	
Acme Tomato Dust	Arsenic	(122)	
Acme Weed Killer	Arsenic	(122)	
Acrylon Spot Fumigant	Carbon Tetrachloride	(124)	
Aero Cyanamid	Cyanamid	(125)	see Cyanide
AFKO	Benzocaine	(125)	see Cocaine
	Phenol	(131)	
	Mercury	(129)	
Agarol	Phenolphthalein	(141)	
Agicide Rat Track	Antu	(121)	
Agicide Spray Base	Rotenone	(133)	
Air-Flo Green	Arsenic	(122)	
Alco	Arsenic	(122)	
Alka Seltzer	Salicylates	(141)	

*Numbers in parentheses refer to pages on which the treatment of the individual poisons is outlined.

The agents marked with an asterisk (*) are generally those which are either inert or those for which no specific therapy is necessary or available.

APPENDIX TABLE I. COMMERCIAL SOURCES OF POISONS—CONT'D

Allonal	Amidopyrine	(138)	
	Barbiturates	(135)	
Alphebin	Amidopyrine	(138)	
	Barbiturates	(135)	
Amidoneonal	Amidopyrine	(138)	
	Barbiturates	(135)	
Ammonia Water	Ammonium Hydroxide	(116, 118, 119)	see Acids and Alkalies
Anacin	Amidopyrine	(138)	
	Barbiturates	(135)	
Analax	Phenolphthalein	(141)	
Anesthesin	Benzocaine	(125)	
	Boric Acid	(122)	
Anhydrous Rasorite	Sodium Borate	(122)	see Boric Acid
Ant-B-gon	Arsenic	(122)	
Anticonvulsants	Bromides	(128)	see Iodine
	Barbiturates	(135)	
	Hydantoin Derivatives	(135)	see Barbiturates
Antifreeze	Ethyl Alcohol	(236)	
	Ethanol	(130)	see Methyl Alcohol
Antimite	Arsenic	(122)	
	Sodium Fluoride	(127)	
Antipyretics	Salicylates	(141)	
Ant paste	Arsenic	(122)	
Ant powder	Pyrethrum	(133)	
Antrol Ant Killer	Arsenic	(122)	
Antrol Ant Syrup	Arsenic	(122)	
Antrol Ant Traps	Arsenic	(122)	
Antu-Alpha Naphthylthiourea	Thallium	(134)	
Ant-X	Thallium	(134)	
Ant-X Jelly Bait	Thallium	(134)	

Appendix Table I. Commercial Sources of Poisons—Cont'd

Apoinite	Rotenone	(133)	
Arab Ant Chips	Arsenic	(122)	
Arab Liquid Rat and Mouse Killer	Arsenic	(122)	
Arab Mothproof	Arsenic	(122)	
Arab Mouse Lure	Strychnine	(142)	
Arab Roach Powder	Fluoride Pyrethrins	(127) (133)	
Argentine Ant Poison	Arsenic	(122)	
Asthma Remedies	Ephedrine Barbiturates Newer Antihis-taminics	(139) (135) (137)	
Atlas A	Arsenic	(122)	
Atlas Cattle Dip	Arsenic	(122)	
Atophan	Cinchophen	(138)	see Benzene Derivatives
Awinc	Pyrethrum	(133)	
Barbak	Mercury Cyanamid	(129) (125)	 see Cyanide
Basi-Cop Dust #3 and #4	Copper Arsenic	(142) (122)	see Zinc Sulfate
Battery Boxes	Lead	(128)	
B.C.A.	Copper Arsenic	(142) (122)	see Zinc Sulfate
B.C.A. with Sulfur	Copper Arsenic Sulfur	(142) (122)	see Zinc Sulfate
Bee Brand Ant and Flea Killer	Rotenone	(133)	
Bee Brand Flea and Tick Killer	DDT	(126)	
Bee Brand Insect Powder	Pyrethrin	(133)	
Bee Brand Roach Killer	DDT Pyrethrin	(126) (133)	

Appendix Table I. Commercial Sources of Poisons—Cont'd

Beinex	Thymol	(131)	see Phenol
	Menthol	(141)	see Salicylates
	Sodium Thiosulfate	(133)	see Sodium Hyposulfite
Benzedo Compound Capsules	Amidopyrine	(138)	
	Barbiturates	(135)	
Benzol	Benzene	(138)	
Berako	Rotenone	(133)	
B H C Magical	Arsenic	(122)	
Bi-Cal	Mercury	(129)	
Bichloride	Mercury	(129)	
Black Flag Flea and Louse Powder	DDT	(126)	
Black Flag Insect Spray	DDT	(126)	
Black Flag Powder	DDT	(126)	
Black Flag Super Insect Spray	DDT	(126)	
	Pyrethrins	(133)	
Black Leaf 40	Nicotine	(130)	
Black Leaf 155	Nicotine	(130)	
Black Leaf Dry Concentrate	Nicotine	(130)	
Black Leaf Garden Dust	Nicotine	(130)	
	Rotenone	(133)	
	Pyrethrum	(133)	
Blue Death Rat Poison Paste	Phosphorus	(132)	
Bonrate	Rotenone	(133)	
Barekil	Nicotine	(130)	
Bowl Clean	Hydrochloric acid	(116)	(118) (119) see Acids and Alkalies
Bridgeport Aer-A-Sol	Pyrethrum	(133)	
Bromidia	Bromides	(128)	see Iodine

Appendix Table I. Commercial Sources of Poisons—Cont'd

Brown Patch Formula	Mercury	(129)	
Brown Rat Poison	Antu	(121)	
Bug Ded	DDT	(126)	
Buhach Insect Powder	Pyrethrins	(133)	
Butyn	Cocaine Derivatives	(125)	
Cabbage Maggot Destroyer	Mercury	(129)	
Calgesic	Benzocaine	(125)	see Cocaine
	Calamine	(142)	see Zinc Sulfate
Calgreen	Arsenic	(122)	
Calinitol	Chloral	(138)	
	Ethanol	(130)	see Methyl Alcohol
	Ether	(135)	see Barbiturates
	Menthol	(141)	see Salicylates
	Camphor	(123)	
Calo-Chlor	Mercury	(129)	
Calogreen	Mercury	(129)	
Caloten	Phenol	(131)	
	Calamine	(142)	see Zinc Sulfate
	Zinc Oxide	(142)	see Zinc Sulfate
Cal-O-Zin	Phenol	(131)	
	Calamine	(142)	see Zinc Sulfate
	Zinc Oxide	(142)	see Zinc Sulfate
Campho-Phenique	Phenol	(131)	
	Camphor	(123)	
Camphor Oil	Camphor	(123)	
Capsules, Reducing	Thyroid	(*)	
	Dinitrophenol	(*)	
	Benzedrine	(138)	
Carbola Copper Dust	Copper	(142)	see Zinc Sulfate
	Rotenone	(133)	

APPENDIX TABLE I. COMMERCIAL SOURCES OF POISONS—CONT'D

Carbola Disinfecting White Paint	Phenol	(131)	
Carbola Garden Dust and Spray	DDT	(126)	
Carbolated Salve	Phenol	(131)	
Carbolic Acid	Phenol	(131)	
Carbona	Carbon Tetrachloride	(124)	
Cascara (Hinkle's)	Atropine Strychnine	(134) (142)	
Casco	Pyrethrin	(133)	
Catex	Phenol	(131)	
Cattle dip	Arsenic	(122)	
C C C Louse Killer	Rotenone	(133)	
Cereson	Mercury	(129)	
Chalk, Colored	Lead	(128)	
Chipinan Parris Green	Arsenic	(122)	
Chipinan Tomato Dust	Arsenic	(122)	
Chlorasol Fumigant	Carbon Tetrachloride	(124)	
Cibalgine	Amidopyrine Barbiturates	(138) (135)	
Cigars	Nicotine	(130)	
Cinchopyrine	Amidopyrine Barbiturates	(138) (135)	
Citro-Mulsion	Hydrocarbon Oil	(138)	see Benzene Derivatives
Cleaners, Metallic	Oxalic Acid Other Acids	(131) (116)	 (118) (119) see Acids and Alkalies
Cleaners, Toilet	Acid Sodium Bisulfate	(116) (133)	(118) (119) see Acids and Alkalies see Sodium Hyposulfite

Appendix Table I. Commercial Sources of Poisons—Cont'd

Cleaners, Pipe and Drain	Alkali	(116)	(118) (119) see Acids and Alkalies
Clinitest	Copper	(142)	see Zinc Sulfate
Clorox	Sodium Hypochlorite	(133)	see Sodium Hyposulfite
Coal Oil	Kerosene	(128)	
Cold Remedies	Aconite Salicylic Acid	(236) (141)	
Cold Wave Neutralizer	Potassium Bromate	(132)	
College Brand Powdered Insecticide	DDT Pyrethrins	(126) (133)	
Cologne Water	Ethyl Alcohol	(236)	
Compound 1080	Sodium Fluoroacetate	(127)	see Fluorides
Cooking, Galvanized Pots	Zinc	(142)	
Cooper's Sheep Dipping Powder	Arsenic	(122)	
Copar	Copper	(128)	
Copper Hydro "C" Dust	Arsenic	(122)	
Cormatal	Resorcinol Zinc Oxide Boric Acid Sodium Thiosulfate	(131) (142) (122) (133)	see Phenol see Zinc Sulfate
Corona Dust Numbers 12, 20, 30, 37, 57, 75, 100, 402, 520, 720	Arsenic	(122)	
Corona Oats Dust	Formaldehyde	(127)	
Corona Southern Peach Dust	Arsenic	(122)	
Corrosive Sublimate	Mercury	(129)	

APPENDIX TABLE I. COMMERCIAL SOURCES OF POISONS—CONT'D

Cough Remedies	Morphine	(140)	
	Codeine	(140)	
	Chloroform	(135)	see Barbiturates
	Opium Derivatives and Related Synthetic Compounds	(140)	
	Antihistaminics	(137)	
	Sulfonamides	(39)	see Anuria
	Ephedrine Sulfate and Related Compounds	(139)	
	Sodium Citrate	(46)	see Alkalosis
	Ammonium Chloride	(28)	see Acidosis
	Antibiotics	(*)	
Cross Country Insect Bait	Arsenic	(122)	
Crystal Borer	Emulsified Naphthalene	(130)	
Cuke and Melon Dust	Arsenic	(122)	
Curran Moth Balls and Flakes	Naphthalene	(130)	
Cut Worm Bait	Arsenic	(122)	
D-50 Dust	DDT	(126)	
D-50 Wettable Powder	DDT	(126)	
D and P Fruit Spray	DDT	(126)	
D and P Tomato Dust	Copper	(128)	
	Arsenic	(122)	
D & P Weed Killer	Arsenic	(122)	
D D-Ide Garden Spray Concentrate	DDT	(126)	
Deenate 10-X 25 R, 25 W, 50 P, 50 W	DDT	(126)	
Dendrol	Petroleum Oil	(128)	

Appendix Table I. Commercial Sources of Poisons—Cont'd

Dental Drugs	Cocaine and Related Drugs	(125)	
Depilatories	Thallium Aluminum Sulfate	(134) (*)	
Derma-Dyne	Phenol Tannin	(131) (*)	
Derma-Medicone	Benzocaine Ephedrine Sulfate	(125) (139)	see Cocaine
Derris Powder	Rotenone	(133)	
Desitin	Zinc Oxide	(142)	see Zinc Sulfate
Devex	DDT	(126)	
Di-Chor-Mulsion	Ethylene Dichloride	(*)	
Diweevil	Carbon Tetrachloride	(124)	
Dolge Weed Killer	Arsenic	(122)	
Domebro Tablets	Aluminum Sulfate Calcium Acetate	(*) (*)	
Dormant Spray Oil	Petroleum Oils	(128)	
Dowfume EB-5, EB-15, 50, G, 75	Carbon Tetrachloride	(124)	
Dow Rose Dust	Arsenic	(122)	
Dow Special Garden Spray	Arsenic	(122)	
Dow Special Potato Spray	Arsenic	(122)	
Drain Cleaners	Lye	(129)	
Draino	Lye	(129)	
Dustrend Roach Powder	Pyrethrum	(133)	
Dwin Insect Killer	Pyrethrum	(133)	
Dye (Shoe)	Aniline	(121)	
Dytox 10	DDT	(126)	
Eagle Spirits	Methyl Alcohol	(130)	
Eastern States Dust Numbers 2, 3, 5	Arsenic	(122)	

APPENDIX TABLE I. COMMERCIAL SOURCES OF POISONS—CONT'D

Eastern States Dust-12	Calomel	(129)	see Mercury
Eastern States Spray A	DDT	(126)	
Eastern States Spray D	Nicotine	(130)	
Eastern States Spray J	DDT	(126)	
El Rey Mouse Bait	Strychnine	(142)	
Emulsion Concentrate	DDT	(126)	
Emulso	Petroleum Oils	(128)	
Enamels	Lead	(128)	
Epidermicide	Salicylic Acid Benzoic Acid Thymol	(141) (*) (131)	 see Phenol
Erl—31, 38	Nicotine	(130)	
Evictor 5 Lb. Cattle Bomb	DDT	(126)	
Ex-Lax	Phenolphthalein	(141)	
Exone	Pine Oil	(*)	
Extox	Phenol Sodium Thiosulfate Camphor Isopropanol	(131) (133) (123) (130)	 see Sodium Hyposulfite see Methyl Alcohol
Extrax Insect Spray	Petroleum Oils	(128)	
Eye Wash	Boric Acid Zinc Sulfate	(122) (142)	
Faesy & Besthoff Tobacco Dust	Nicotine	(130)	
Faesy & Besthoff Weed Killer	Arsenic	(122)	

Appendix Table I. Commercial Sources of Poisons—Cont'd

Fairmount Weed Killer	Arsenic	(122)	
Falcon Roach Powder	Pyrethrins Sodium Fluoride	(133) (127)	
Farm Bureau General Purpose Spray	Arsenic	(122)	
Farm Bureau Potato Spray	Copper DDT	(142) (126)	see Zinc Sulfate
Farm Master Lice Powder	Sodium Fluoride	(127)	
Farm Master Livestock Fly Spray	Pyrethrum	(133)	
Farmrite Cucurbit Dust	Arsenic	(122)	
Farmrite Orchard Mouse Bait	Strychnine	(142)	
Farmrite Paris Green	Arsenic	(122)	
Farmrite Potato & Tomato Spray	Arsenic	(122)	
Farmrite Triple Peach Spray	Arsenic	(122)	
Farmrite Tomato Dust with Poison	Arsenic	(122)	
Fire Blight Disinfectant	Mercurial	(129)	
Fireworks	Mercury Phosphorus	(129) (132)	
Devil on the Walk	Phosphorus	(132)	
Giant Torpedoes	Phosphorus	(132)	
Pharaoh's Serpent	Mercury	(129)	
Snake in the Grass	Mercury	(129)	
Son-of-a-Gun	Phosphorus	(132)	
Flea Powder	Rotenone	(133)	
Flight	Naphthalene	(130)	

APPENDIX TABLE I. COMMERCIAL SOURCES OF POISONS—CONT'D

Flo-Mulsion	Hydrocarbon Oils	(128)
Floridoil	Hydrocarbon Oils	(128)
Fly Funineral	DDT Kerosene	(126) (128)
Fly Gas	Pyrethrum	(133)
Fly Paper	Arsenic	(122)
Foille	Phenol	(131)
Formalin	Formaldehyde	(127)
Fowler's Solution	Arsenic	(122)
Free Mulsion	Petroleum Oils	(128)
Fresnol Antjar	Arsenic	(122)
Froth Liquid Moth Spray	Carbon Tetrachloride	(124)
Fuel Lighter Fluid Spirits Canned Heat "Sterno"	 Hydrocarbons Ethyl or Methyl Alcohol Alcohol	 (128) (130) (236) (238) (130)
Fuedeth Roach Powder	Sodium Fluoride	(127)
Fume-Rite	Nicotine	(130)
Furniture Polish	Lemon Oil Kerosene-like Volatile Hydrocarbons	(*) (128)
Garden Dust	Arsenic	(122)
Garden Master Potato Spray	DDT	(126)
Geigy's Potato Vine and Weed Killer	Arsenic	(122)
General Chemical Tobacco Dust	Nicotine	(130)
General Chemical 668	Mercury	(129)

Appendix Table I. Commercial Sources of Poisons—Cont'd

Genitol EM-25	DDT	(126)	
Gesarol S-30	DDT	(126)	
VD-50	DDT	(126)	
Gildings	Benzene	(138)	
Gland-O-Lac Roost Spread	Nicotine	(130)	
Glazes	Lead	(128)	
"Gopher-Go"	Strychnine	(142)	
Greenol	Petroleum Oil	(128)	
Grub-O	Arsenic	(122)	
Gta Ant Bone	Thallium	(134)	
Gta Bait for Rats	Thallium	(134)	
Gulfspray Roach and Ant Killer	Pyrethrins	(133)	
Gulf Trak	DDT	(126)	
Gypsy	Phenol	(131)	
	Zinc Oxide	(142)	see Zinc Sulfate
	Camphor	(123)	
Halowax	Naphthalene	(130)	
Hammonds Weed Killer	Arsenic	(122)	
Handy Killer	Arsenic	(122)	
Hat (Straw) Cleaners	Oxalic Acid	(131)	
Headache powders	Amidopyrine	(138)	
	Salicylates	(141)	
	Caffeine	(138)	see Benzedrine
	Dexedrine	(138)	
Hinkle's Cascara	Strychnine	(142)	
	Atropine	(134)	
Holly Pipe Cleaner	Lye	(129)	
Hort Spray	DDT	(126)	
Ice, Camphor	Camphor	(123)	
Ice, Dry	CO_2 Snow	(*)	

APPENDIX TABLE I. COMMERCIAL SOURCES OF POISONS—CONT'D

Imp. Soap Spray	Nicotine	(130)	
Infuco Grain Fumigant	Carbon Tetrachloride	(124)	
Infuco 80-20 Grain Fumigant	Carbon Tetrachloride	(124)	
	Carbon Disulfide	(123)	
Infuco Rodenticide	Arsenic	(122)	
Infuco Sectocide	Ethylene Dichloride	(236)	
	Carbon Tetrachloride	(124)	
Inhalers	Benzedrine and Related Derivatives	(138)	
	Menthol	(141)	see Salicylates
	Sympathicomimetic Drugs	(139)	see Ephedrine
Ink, Marking	Silver Salts	(133)	
Iritex	Phenol	(131)	
	Zinc Oxide	(142)	see Zinc Sulfate
	Camphor	(123)	
Ivy	Belladonna	(134)	
	Magnesium Sulfate	(237)	
	Sodium Thiosulfate	(133)	see Sodium Hyposulfite
	Menthol	(141)	see Salicylates
Ivy-Chek	Ferric Chloride	(139)	see Iron
I-V-Eze	Phenol	(131)	
	Calamine	(142)	see Zinc Sulfate
Ivy Dry	Tannic Acid	(*)	
Ivolav	Sodium Thiosulfate	(133)	see Sodium Hyposulfite
	Acetone	(*)	
Ivolon	Magnesium Sulfate	(237)	
	Boric Acid	(122)	
	Acetic Acid	(116)	(118) (119) see Acids and Alkalies
Ivy-Go	Phenol	(131)	
	Zinc Oxide	(142)	see Zinc Sulfate
	Camphor	(123)	

Appendix Table I. Commercial Sources of Poisons—Cont'd

Ivy-Tox	Cresol Lead Subacetate	(131) (128)	
J-O Roach-Rat Paste	Phosphorus	(132)	
Jimson Weed	Atropine	(134)	
Keenup Dormant Oil	Petroleum Oil	(128)	
Kemicide Spray	Pyrethrum	(133)	
Kero-Kill	Pyrethrum	(133)	
Kero-Kill Special	Pyrethrum Carbon Tetrachloride	(133) (124)	
Kleenup Soluble Dormant Oil Spray	Petroleum Oil	(128)	
Knox Out Stock & Barn Spray	DDT	(126)	
Kolokil	Arsenic	(122)	
Kolotex	Arsenic	(122)	
Krop-Saver D C Vegetable Spray	Copper DDT	(142) (126)	see Zinc Sulfate
Krop Saver 25 DE	DDT	(126)	
Krop Saver Dust Numbers 5, 10, 75	Pyrethrin	(133)	
Kryax	Sodium Fluoride	(127)	
Kryocide	Sodium Fluoaluminate	(127)	see Fluorides
Krytox	Sodium Fluoaluminate	(127)	see Fluorides
Laudanum	Morphine and Derivatives	(140)	
Liverty Weed Tox	Arsenic	(122)	
Liquid Moth Proofer	Sodium Silicofluoride	(127)	
Lotions, Teething	Opium Derivatives Mercury Benzocaine and Derivatives	(140) (129) (125)	 see Cocaine

APPENDIX TABLE I. COMMERCIAL SOURCES OF POISONS—CONT'D

Lugol's Solution	Iodine	(128)	
Luminous Paints	Phosphorus Radium	(132) (*)	
Lye	Strong Alkali	(116)	(118) (119) see Acids and Alkalies
Lysol	Phenol Derivatives	(131)	
Mackoblend Spray	DDT	(126)	
Mackopray	DDT	(126)	
Magikil Jelly Ant Bait	Thallium Sulfate	(134)	
Matches	Phosphorus	(132)	
Mazon Ointment	Benzoic Acid Salicylic Acid Tars Mercury Salicylate Sodium Stearate	(*) (141) (*) (141) (*)	 see Salicylates
Mechling's Ant Killer	DDT	(126)	
Mechling's Paris Green	Arsenic	(122)	
Mentholatum	Menthol	(141)	see Salicylates
Mersolite	Mercury	(129)	
Mersolite 8	Mercury	(129)	
Merthiolate	Mercury	(129)	
Midol	Amidopyrine Barbiturates	(138) (135)	
Millerfume	Carbon Bisulphide	(123)	see Carbon Disulfide
Miller's Household Dust	DDT	(126)	
Miller's Gardusto	Arsenic Copper Nicotine	(122) (142) (130)	 see Zinc Sulfate
Miller's Weed Killer	Arsenic	(122)	

Appendix Table I. Commercial Sources of Poisons—Cont'd

Mill-O-Cide Concentrate	Pyrethrum	(133)	
Mirbone	Aniline	(121)	
Mist Air	Pyrethrum	(133)	
Mon-O-Spray	Rotenone	(133)	
Mop-N-Mix	Arsenic	(122)	
Moth Balls and Powder	Naphthalene	(130)	
Mothend Moth Spray	Pyrethrum	(133)	
Mothicide Moth Killer	Carbon Tetrachloride	(124)	
Moth	Carbon Tetrachloride	(124)	
Moth Spray	Pyrethrum	(133)	
Mulch-Rite	Nicotine	(130)	
Mylin	Amidopyrine Barbiturates	(138) (135)	
Nasal Sprays	Ephedrine and Related Compounds Menthol Cocaine and Related Compounds Antihistaminics Sulfonamides Antibiotics Silver Salts	(139) (141) (125) (137) (39) (*) (133)	 see Salicylates see Anuria
Neonal	Amidopyrine Barbiturates	(138) (135)	
New Improved Cereson	Mercury	(129)	
Nico-Fume Liquid	Nicotine	(130)	
Nico-Mulsion	Nicotine Petroleum Oils	(130) (128)	
Nicotrox-10-X	Nicotine	(130)	
Nicotrol	Nicotine	(130)	

Appendix Table I. Commercial Sources of Poisons—Cont'd

Nip-An-Tuck Roach Powder	Pyrethrins	(133)	
	Sodium Fluoride	(127)	
Nipple Shields	Lead	(128)	
Nitrobenzene	Aniline Group	(121)	
No. 6 Paste Rat and Mouse Controller	Thallium	(134)	
Nomad	Phenol	(131)	
	Zinc Oxide	(142)	see Zinc Sulfate
	Camphor	(123)	
Nyderma	Phenol	(131)	
	Methyl Salicylate	(141)	
Oil, Camphorated	Camphor	(123)	
Oil, Coal Oil	Kerosene	(128)	
Oil, Mirbane	Aniline	(121)	
Oil, Wintergreen	Methyl Salicylate	(141)	
Oil Tone	Petroleum Oil	(128)	
O.K. Plant Spray	Nicotine	(130)	
Omnicide B B	DDT	(126)	
	Pyrethrum	(133)	
One Eighty (180)	Copper	(142)	see Zinc Sulfate
	Arsenic	(122)	
O-N	Salicylic Acid	(141)	
	Benzoic Acid	(*)	
Orbiscide Cube Powder	Rotenone	(133)	
Orchard Brand Paris Green	Arsenic	(122)	
Ormont	Aluminum Sulfate and Hydroxide	(*)	
Orthodinitrobenzol	Aniline Group	(121)	
Orthol-D Emulsion	Petroleum Oils	(128)	
Orthol-D Soluble	Petroleum Oils	(128)	
Orthol Garden Spray	Nicotine	(130)	
	Petroleum Oils	(128)	

APPENDIX TABLE I. COMMERCIAL SOURCES OF POISONS—CONT'D

Out-Weed Weed Killer	Arsenic	(122)	
Out-Weed XX Weed Killer	Arsenic	(122)	
Paint	Lead	(128)	
Paint Remover	Alcohols	(130)	
Pan Apple Spray	Arsenic	(122)	
	Copper	(142)	see Zinc Sulfate
	Zinc	(142)	
Pan Peach Spray	Arsenic	(122)	
	Sulfur	(*)	
	Zinc	(142)	
Pan Plant Spray	Arsenic	(122)	
	Copper	(128)	
	Nicotine	(130)	
	Sulfur	(*)	
Paris Green	Arsenic	(122)	
Parsons Cal-C-Note	Arsenic	(122)	
Parsons Smut-Off Solution	Formaldehyde	(127)	
	Mercury	(129)	
Paste, Ant	Arsenic	(122)	
Paste, Solder	Zinc	(142)	
Penco Cattle Spray	DDT	(126)	
Penite	Arsenic	(122)	
Peralga	Amidopyrine	(138)	
	Barbiturates	(135)	
Peraminal	Amidopyrine	(138)	
	Barbiturates	(135)	
Persisto Wettable	DDT	(126)	
Pest-B-Gon Spray	DDT	(126)	
Pestmaster Easy Emulsifying Concentrate	DDT	(126)	
	Petroleum Oils	(128)	
Pestmaster Tomato Dust	Arsenic	(122)	

Appendix Table I. Commercial Sources of Poisons—Cont'd

Peterman Flea Powder	Pyrethrins	(133)	
Peterman Roach Powder & Paste	Sodium Fluoride	(127)	
Pharaoh's Serpent	Mercury	(129)	
Phenola	Phenolphthalein	(141)	
Photographer's Solution	Sodium Hyposulfite Silver Salts	(133) (133)	
Plant-Rite 75, 100	Nicotine	(130)	
P.M.A.S.	Mercury	(129)	
Poison Ivy Wash	Ferric Chloride	(139)	see Iron
Potato Copar	Arsenic Copper	(122) (142)	 see Zinc Sulfate
Potato Dust	Arsenic Copper	(122) (142)	 see Zinc Sulfate
Potato Powder #1	Arsenic Copper	(122) (142)	 see Zinc Sulfate
Potato Spray	Arsenic Copper	(122) (142)	 see Zinc Sulfate
Powders, Anti-convulsants (or Tablets)	Barbiturates Bromides Dilantin Mesantoin Tridione and Related Drugs	(135) (128) (135) (135) (142)	 see Iodine see Barbiturates see Barbiturates
Pratt's Fruit Tree Spray	Arsenic	(122)	
Prentox Micro Mesh Dry	DDT	(126)	
Pronto	Lye	(129)	
Protex	Arsenic Copper	(122) (142)	 see Zinc Sulfate
Purex (Bleach)	Sodium Hypochlorite	(133)	
Purex Pipe and Drain Cleaner	Lye	(129)	

Appendix Table I. Commercial Sources of Poisons—Cont'd

Putty	Lead	(128)	
Pyrox	Arsenic	(122)	
	Copper	(142)	see Zinc Sulfate
Pyrene (Fire Extinguisher)	Carbon Tetrachloride	(124)	
R.A.B.	Pyrethrins	(133)	
	DDT	(126)	
Rat Poison	Strychnine	(142)	
	Arsenic	(122)	
	Copper	(142)	see Zinc Sulfate
	Thallium	(134)	
	Phosphorus	(132)	
	Fluorides	(127)	
	Cyanide	(125)	
Red Arrow Garden Spray	Pyrethrins	(133)	
Red Arrow D-10 Louse Powder	DDT	(126)	
Red Arrow D-25 Orchid Spray	DDT	(126)	
Red Arrow D-50 Water Dispersible Powder	DDT	(126)	
Red River Potato Mix	Copper	(142)	see Zinc Sulfate
	DDT	(126)	
Resinol	Resorcinol	(131)	see Phenol
	Calamine	(142)	see Zinc Sulfate
	Bismuth Subnitrate	(138)	
	Zinc Oxide	(142)	see Zinc Sulfate
Resin Solvents	Naphthalene	(130)	
Restix Emulsifiable & Concentrate Insecticide	DDT	(126)	
Rex Roach Powder	Pyrethrins	(133)	

APPENDIX TABLE I. COMMERCIAL SOURCES OF POISONS—CONT'D

Rhulital	Phenol Tannic Acid Camphor Boric Acid	(131) (*) (123) (122)	
Roach Bate	Sodium Borate	(122)	see Boric Acid
Roach Cafe	Sodium Borate	(122)	see Boric Acid
Roach Ded	DDT	(126)	
Roach Killer	DDT	(126)	
Roach-End Roach Spray	Pyrethrum	(133)	
Roach Powder	Sodium Fluoride	(127)	
Ro-Ko	Rotenone	(133)	
Safite Roach Powder	Pyrethrum Sodium Fluoride	(133) (127)	
Saftifume Briquette	Cyanogen Chloride	(125)	see Cyanide
Dr. Salisbury's Nic-Sol	Nicotine	(130)	
Sanaseed Impregnated Bird Seed	Strychnine	(142)	
Sani-Flush	Sodium Bisulfate	(133)	see Sodium Hyposulfite
Santobane-50	DDT	(126)	
Scaloyl	Petroleum Oils	(128)	
Sheep Dip	Phenols	(131)	
Skalekut	Lye	(129)	
Sloan's Liniment	Camphor	(123)	
Snail Killer	Methaldehyde	(138)	see Benzene Derivatives
Snaral	Arsenic Methaldehyde	(122) (138)	 see Benzene Derivatives
New Snaral	Methaldehyde *only*	(138)	see Benzene Derivatives
"Snow"	Cocaine	(125)	

APPENDIX TABLE I. COMMERCIAL SOURCES OF POISONS—CONT'D

Snowflake Moth Spray	Carbon Tetrachloride	(124)	
Soldering Paste	Zinc	(142)	
Soldering Solution	Acid	(116)	(118) (119) see Acids and Alkalis
Southern States 620 Dust	Arsenic Copper	(122) (142)	 see Zinc Sulfate
Spot Remover	Hydrofluoric Acid	(127)	
Sproof Moth Proofer	Sodium Silicofluoride	(127)	
Stern's Electric Paste Rat Poison	Phosphorus Arsenic	(132) (122)	
Strawberry Dust	Sulfur	(*)	
Sublimate, Corrosive	Mercury	(129)	
Sulphur Lead Dusts	Sulfur Lead Arsenic	(*) (128) (122)	
Surfacaine	Cyclomethycaine	(125)	see Cocaine
S.W. Paris Green	Arsenic	(122)	
Syndeet, 30; S 30; 50 W	DDT	(126)	
Tabro Roach Tablets	Boric Acid Borax	(122) (122)	 see Boric Acid
T A T Ant Bait	Thallium	(134)	
T A T Ant Trap	Thallium	(134)	
T A T Mo-Go	Thallium	(134)	
T A T Soilicide	Mercury	(129)	
T A T 30% Solution Concentrate	DDT	(126)	
Teething Lotion	Morphine and Related Compounds Benzocaine and Related Compounds Mercury	(140) (125) (129)	 see Cocaine

Appendix Table I. Commercial Sources of Poisons—Cont'd

Tendust	Nicotine	(130)	
Tetralin	Naphthalene	(130)	
Thalgrain	Thallium	(134)	
Thyptal	Phenol Kaolin Alumina Gel	(131) (*) (*)	
Toilet Bowl Clean	Sodium Bisulfite Acids Lye	(133) (116) (129)	 (118) (119) see Acids and Alkalis
Tomato Copar Dust Tomato Dust Tomato Powder	Arsenic Copper	(122) (142)	 see Zinc Sulfate
Toni Home Permanent (Cold Wave Neutralizer)	Potassium Bromate	(132)	
Tree Fumigation	Cyanide	(125)	
Triclane Dust	DDT	(126)	
Trikal	Copper Arsenic	(142) (122)	see Zinc Sulfate
Triox	Arsenic	(122)	
Tri-Spray	Copper Nicotine	(142) (130)	see Zinc Sulfate
Turpentine	Turpentine	(134)	
Twenty X-N	Nicotine	(130)	
Twin Light Arsocop	Arsenic Copper	(122) (142)	 see Zinc Sulfate
Twin Light Cabbage Root Dust	Calomel	(129)	see Mercury
Twin Light Despray	DDT	(126)	
University Brand Grain Fumigant	Carbon Tetrachloride	(124)	
Usanigas 1	Carbon Tetrachloride	(124)	
Varnish	Alcohols	(130)	

Appendix Table I. Commercial Sources of Poisons—Cont'd

Verdol	Petroleum Oils	(128)	
Vicks	Camphor	(123)	
Vince	Sodium Perborate	(122)	see Boric Acid
Vine Kil	Arsenic	(122)	
Weed Killer	Arsenic	(122)	
Weednox	Arsenic	(122)	
Weedon	Arsenic	(122)	
White Enamel	Arsenic	(122)	
Wilkil	Pyrethrin	(133)	
Wilsonite	Magnesium Arsenate	(122)	see Arsenic
	Copper	(142)	see Zinc Sulfate
	Nicotine	(130)	
Wilson's Weed Killer	Arsenic	(122)	
Wood Alcohol	Methyl Alcohol	(130)	
X-It Rat & Mouse Poison	Arsenic	(122)	
Zema	Phenol	(131)	
	Benzoic Acid	(*)	
	Boric Acid	(122)	
	Potassium Nitrate	(140)	
	Menthol	(141)	see Salicylates
	Methyl Salicylate	(141)	
Zonite	Sodium Hypochlorite	(133)	see Sodium Hyposulfite
	Sodium Hydroxide	(116)	(118) (119) see Acids and Alkalis
	Sodium Chloride	(*)	
Zotox	Arsenic	(122)	

APPENDIX TABLE II. POISONS GENERALLY FOUND IN HOUSEHOLD ARTICLES*

Antiseptics	Boric Acid	(122)	
	Bichloride of Mercury	(129)	
	Formaldehyde	(127)	
	Iodine	(128)	
	Phenols	(131)	
	Silver Nitrate	(133)	
Asthma Remedies	Aminophylline	(236)	
	Antihistamines	(137)	
	Atropine	(134)	
	Barbiturates	(135)	
	Ephedrine and Related Compounds	(139)	
	Iodine	(128)	
Athlete's Foot Medications	Copper Salts	(142)	see Zinc Sulfate
	Formaldehyde	(127)	
	Iodine	(128)	
	Merthiolate	(129)	see Mercury
	Phenol	(131)	
	Salicylic Acid	(141)	
	Sodium Hypochlorite	(133)	see Sodium Hyposulfite
Baby Powder	Zinc Stearate	(238)	
Bleaching Agents	Acetic Acid	(116)	(118) (119) see Acids and Alkalis
	Hydrogen Peroxide	(*)	
	Oxalates	(131)	
	Sodium Hypochlorite	(133)	see Sodium Hyposulfite
Cigarette Lighter Fluid	Benzene Derivatives	(138)	

*Numbers in parentheses refer to pages on which the treatment of the individual poisons is outlined.

The agents marked with an asterisk (*) are generally those which are either inert or those for which no specific therapy is necessary or available.

Appendix Table II. Poisons Generally Found in Household Articles—Cont'd

Cleaning Solutions	Alkalis	(116) (118) (119) see Acids and Alkalis
	Ammonia Water	(116) (118) (119) see Acids and Alkalis
	Benzene Derivatives	(138)
	Carbon Tetrachloride	(124)
	Cyanides	(125)
	Kerosene	(128)
	Methyl Alcohol	(130)
	Mineral Acids and Alkalis	(116) (118) (119) see Acids and Alkalis
	Nitric Acid	(116) (118) (119) see Acids and Alkalis
	Oxalic Acid	(131)
	Silver Nitrate	(133)
	Sulfuric Acid	(116) (118) (119) see Acids and Alkalis
Cold Wave Permanents	Potassium Bromate	(132)
Cosmetics	Aniline Derivatives	(121)
	Barium Sulfide	(128) see Lead
	Bismuth	(128) see Lead
	Lead	(128)
	Mercurials	(129)
	Salicylic Acid	(141)
	Silver	(133)
	Sodium Sulfide	(133) see Sodium Hyposulfite
	Sulfur	(*)
	Thallium	(134)

Appendix Table II. Poisons Generally Found in Household Articles—Cont'd

Cough Remedies	Ammonium Chloride	(27) (28) see Acidosis
	Antibiotics	(*)
	Antihistamines	(137)
	Chloroform	(140) see Opiates
	Codeine	(140)
	Ephedrine and Related Compounds	(139)
	Morphine and Related Drugs	(140)
	Sodium Citrate	(46) See Alkalosis
	Sulfonamides	(37) see Anuria
Dyes	Arsenic	(122)
	Benzene Derivatives	(138)
	Heavy Metals	(128) see Lead
Fireworks	Arsenic	(122)
	Mercury	(129)
	Phosphorus	(132)
Inks	Aniline	(121)
	Iron Gallate	(139) see Iron
Indelible Ink	Silver Nitrate	(133)
Ink Removers	Oxalic Acid	(116) (118) (119) see Acids and Alkalis
	Acetic Acid	(131)
Insecticides and Rodenticides	Antu	(121)
	Arsenic	(122)
	Cyanides	(125)
	Dichloricide	(236)
	Dichlorphenol	(236)
	DDT	(126)
	Fluorides	(127)
	Lead	(128)
	Naphthalene	(130)
	Nicotine	(130)
	Phenols	(131)
	Phosphorus	(132)
	Pyrethrum	(133)
	Thallium	(134)

Appendix Table II. Poisons Generally Found in Household Articles—Cont'd

Article	Poison	Ref.	Remarks
Matches	Manganese Dioxide	(*)	
	Potassium Chlorate	(133)	
	Sulfur	(*)	
Metal Polish	Cyanide	(125)	
	Oxalic Acid	(131)	
Ophthalmic Medications	Boric Acid	(122)	
	Heavy Metals	(128)	see Lead
	Parasympathicomimetic Drugs	(139)	see Mecholyl
	Sympathicomimetic Drugs	(139)	see Ephedrine
Paints, Paint Removers, Varnishes	Benzene Derivatives	(138)	
	Heavy Metals	(128)	see Lead
	Methyl Alcohol	(130)	
	Turpentine	(134)	
Washing Powders	Borax	(122)	see Boric Acid
	Sodium Carbonate	(116)	(118) (119) see Acids and Alkalis
	Sodium Hypochlorite	(133)	see Sodium Hyposulfite
	Trisodium Phosphate	(116)	(118) (119) see Acids and Alkalis
Waxes (Floor)	Beeswax	(*)	
	Carnauba Wax	(*)	
	Naphtha	(130)	see Naphthalene
	Turpentine	(134)	
Weed Killers	Arsenic	(122)	
	Copper	(142)	see Zinc Sulfate

Appendix Table III. Useful Conversion Methods

1. Factors for the conversion of concentrations expressed in milligram per 100 ml. to milliequivalent per liter:

Calcium	0.4988	Phosphorus (Valence 1)	0.3226
Chloride	0.2817	Phosphorus (Valence 1.8)	0.5814
Magnesium	0.8230	Sodium	0.4348
Potassium	0.2558	Sulfur (Valence 2)	0.625

2. Factor for conversion of volumes per cent to milliequivalents per liter:
   Divide volumes per cent by 2.2

3. Method of changing from milligrams per 100 ml. to milliequivalent per liter:

$$\text{mEq} = \frac{\text{Mg/100 ml.} \times 10}{\text{Valence}}$$

4. Correlation of square meters of body surface with kilogram of body weight for a person of average configuration may be indicated as follows:
   0.5 sq.m. of body surface = 11 kg. of body weight
   1.0 sq.m. of body surface = 28 kg. of body weight
   1.7 sq.m. of body surface = 64 kg. of body weight

APPENDIX TABLE IV. NORMAL PHYSICAL AND CHEMICAL CONSTANTS*

1. Blood Values of Importance in Evaluating States of Dehydration, Electrolyte Disturbance, Acid-Base Balance, etc., and Common Variations in Determinations

DETERMINATION	NORMAL VALUE		VALUE INCREASED	VALUE DECREASED
Calcium (Total serum) Calcium (Ionized in serum)	10.0-12.0 mg./100 c.c. 5.0-5.5 mg./100 c.c.	5.0-6.0 mEq./L.	Acidosis Hyperparathyroidism Pyloric obstruction	Diarrhea (Post-acidotic syndrome) Nephrotic syndrome Oxalic acid poisoning Renal insufficiency Rickets Starvation Tetany (Infantile)
Carbon dioxide content (Serum) Carbon dioxide content (Whole blood)	45-70 vol. % 40-60 vol. %	20.3-31.5 mM/L. 18.0-27.0 mM/L.	Alkali ingestion Aspirin intoxication (Early) Morphine poisoning Pneumonia Vomiting	Acid ingestion Addison's disease Anesthesia Aspirin intoxication (Late) Dehydration Diarrhea Methyl alcohol poisoning Oil of wintergreen poisoning Renal insufficiency Starvation
Chlorides (Serum) expressed as Cl Chlorides (Serum) expressed as NaCl	355-376 mg./100 c.c. 585-620 mg./100 c.c.	100-106 mEq./L. 100-106 mEq./L.	Anesthesia Diuresis due to chloride and sulfate diuretics Hyperventilation Ingestion of chlorides or too rapid administration parenterally of chloride containing solutions—even isotonic saline	Addison's disease Diabetes mellitus Diarrhea Diuresis due to water or mercurials Nephrosis and nephritis Pneumonia Starvation Vomiting
Phosphorus (Inorganic serum) expressed as P	4.5-5.5 mg./100 c.c.	1.45-1.77 mM/L.	Renal insufficiency Rickets	Diabetes Diarrhea Hyperparathyroidism Rickets
Potassium (Serum)	16-22 mg./100 c.c.	4.0-5.5 mEq./L.	Addison's disease Potassium administration Renal insufficiency Shock	Adrenocortical tumor Diarrhea Diabetes (Especially during therapy with alkali or saline) Doca administration Fever Nephrotic syndrome Periodic familial paralysis

*For practical purposes generally employed in emergency problems, only certain chemical determinations have been selected. Similarly, only those conditions have been included in the last two columns which may, in general, be encountered as emergency problems.

Appendix Table IV. Normal Physical and Chemical Constants—Cont'd

1. Blood Values of Importance in Evaluating States of Dehydration, Electrolyte Disturbance, Acid-Base Balance, etc., and Common Variations in Determinations

DETERMINATION	NORMAL VALUE		VALUE INCREASED	VALUE DECREASED
Sodium (Serum)	307-330 mg./100 c.c.	133-143 mEq./L.	Adrenocortical tumor Cardiac decompensation Doca administration Nephrotic syndrome Renal insufficiency Vomiting	Addison's disease Diabetes mellitus Diarrhea Low sodium diet Nephrotic syndrome Renal insufficiency Starvation Sweating (Excess) Vomiting
Sugar (Fasting, arterial blood) Sugar (Fasting, venous blood) Sugar (Newborn, fasting, venous blood)	80-120 mg./100 c.c. 70-100 mg./100 c.c. 55-75 mg./100 c.c. (Occasionally lower)		Anesthesia Asphyxia Brain injury Cold Diabetes mellitus Excitement Insulin resistance	Acute adrenal insufficiency Hyperinsulinism (Excess insulin administration or insufficient food intake)
Nonprotein nitrogen (Plasma) Nonprotein nitrogen (Whole blood) Urea nitrogen (Plasma) Urea nitrogen (Whole blood)	18-30 mg./100 c.c. 25-40 mg./100 c.c. 14-32 mg./100 c.c. 7-15 mg./100 c.c.		Cardiac decompensation Dehydration Diarrhea Fever Hemorrhage Renal insufficiency Shock	Diuresis Starvation
	(Gm./100 ml.)			
Total proteins (Plasma) Premature infant Full term infant Birth to 1 yr. 1 to 4 yr. 5 to 12 yr. 12 yr. and over	 4.55 ± 0.59 5.11 – 5.70 6.10 ± 0.29 6.49 ± 0.47 7.30 ± 0.59 7.16		Burns Dehydration (With shock) Diarrhea Excess sweating Vomiting	Acute nephritis Blood and plasma loss Cardiac decompensation Chronic intestinal obstruction Liver disease Nephrotic syndrome Starvation
Albumin (Plasma) Premature infant Full term infant Birth to 1 yr. 1 to 4 yr. 5 to 12 yr. 12 yr. and over	 3.55 ± 0.65 3.76 – 3.79 4.97 ± 0.73 4.59 – 4.83 5.0 ± 0.78 4.72		Same as for total proteins	Same as for total proteins
Specific gravity (Whole blood) Newborn	1.048 – 1.050 1.060 – 1.085		Same as for total proteins	Same as for total proteins

Appendix Table IV. Normal Physical and Chemical Constants—Cont'd

2. Miscellaneous Blood Determinations	
Bleeding time	1-3 min.
Coagulation time (Test tube method)	3-9 min.
Prothrombin time (Quick)	12-15 min.
Prothrombin time (Warner)	300 units/c.c. plasma
Lead (Serum)	0.001 to 0.003 mg./100 ml.

3. Normal Cerebrospinal Fluid Values

DETERMINATION	NORMAL VALUE	
Cell count		
Under 1 yr.	0-30 cells/c.mm.	
1 to 4 yr.	20 cells/c.mm.	
5 yr. and over	10 cells/c.mm.	
Chlorides		
7 days to 3 mo.	636-716 mg./100 ml.	108.8-122.5 mEq./L.
4 to 12 mo.	659-742 mg./100 ml.	112.7-128.5 mEq./L.
13 mo. to 12 yr.	683-763 mg./100 ml.	116.8-130.5 mEq./L.
Glucose		
6 mo. to 10 yr.	71-90 mg./100 ml.	
10 yr. and over	50-80 mg./100 ml.	
Protein (Total, lumbar fluid)	15-55 mg./100 ml.	
Albumin	80% of total protein	
Globulin	20% of total protein	
Pandy reaction	Negative	
Lactic acid	Trace (May increase on standing)	

INDEX